DEDICATION

This book is dedicated to:

My Heavenly Father, to thank Him for His guidance; enlightening me enough to put knowledge, wisdom and truth into words; embracing me with His peace; carrying me through the darkness into His light; and above all, loving me unconditionally. Hoping that my soul becomes as perfect as is His Holy Spirit, all I can do is thank Him for loving me.

My Earthly Mother, to thank Her for sustaining my body with fresh air and sunshine, fresh wholesome food to eat, fresh water to drink; surrounding me with Her beauty and joy in every way possible. In return, I promise to honor Her until the end of this earthly life. I thank Her for helping my body to become as perfect as is Her earthly body.

My Earthly Family, a special *"thank you"* to Rolf, Dagmar, Peter, Mom and Dad for challenging me to become all I can possibly be.

Wayne, Jane and Mary Ann, many thanks for refining my German migrant English.

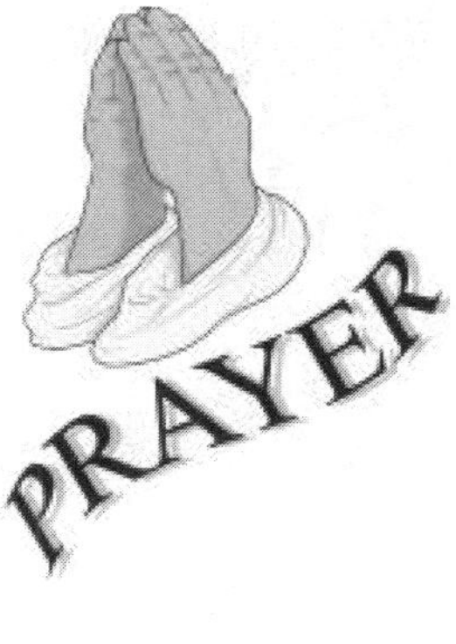

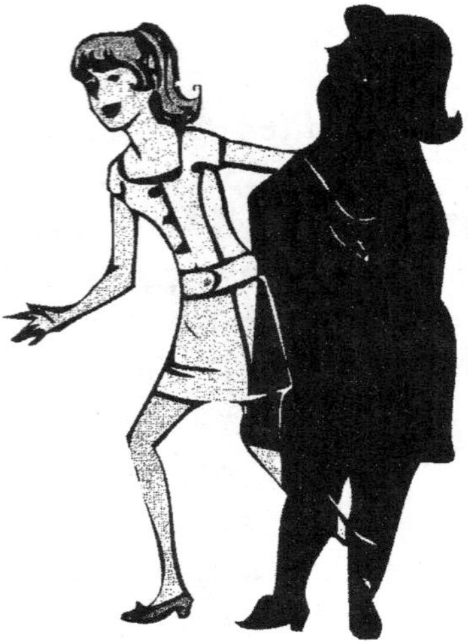

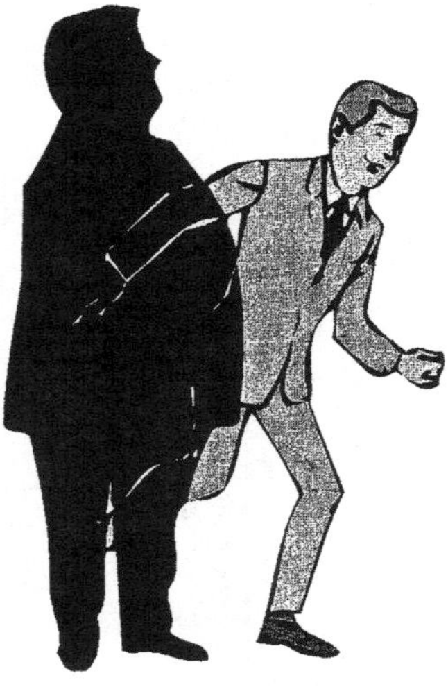

Diets And Why Most Don't Work

Personalizing Your Diet To Suit Your Blood Type And Your Body's Needs

DOB: 1942
Revised edition

Published by:
New Century Press
1055 Bay Boulevard, Suite C
Chula Vista, CA 91911
(800) 519-2465 or (619) 476-7400
www.newcenturypress.com

ISBN 1-890035-21-1

U.S.A. $11.95
CANADA $16.95
First Edition March 1990
Second Revised Edition 2001
Printed on Recycled Paper

In the importance of biochemical individuality, certain truths are self-evident:

- All diets, supplements and medications do not work the same for all people.

- Research indicates that blood type and spiritual awareness can determine nutritional needs.

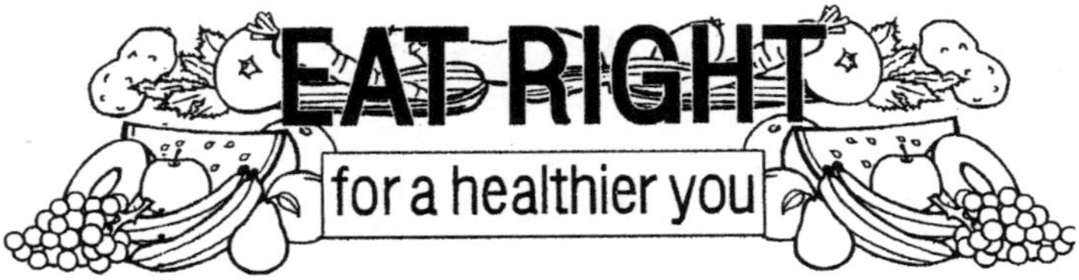

FOREWORD

Most diets don't work and if they do, the weight lost often comes back. During the dieting process a person often becomes sick, tired, disenchanted and then quickly returns to old habits of eating.

Let's define the word "Diet." It's a Greek word meaning a way of life, which indicates one's need to change his/her lifestyle to achieve permanent results.

In my holistic practice of nutritional counseling of overweight people, I have observed that what appeared to work with some did not work for others. I wondered if my findings on blood types would be the missing factor. Further investigation led me to the conclusion that the "Blood Type" of the person makes the difference, especially when each individual's biochemical uniqueness is considered.

Another factor to consider might be a deep-seated emotional problem such as child/spouse abuse, loss of a loved one, or just feeling unloved or lonely.

In general, food temporarily comforts and makes one feel better for a while. But every time a person feels hurt or depressed, they tend to eat to comfort the child within, and a vicious cycle begins.

Research indicates that children who were breast-fed usually are not overweight later in life. The hormone oxytoxin, a part of mother's milk, helps to make babies feel good, comforted and calm, while providing them with a sense of belonging.

The same hormone is also released when one is in love, making love or eating. Now at least we know why "food" in general makes us feel good.

It is important for our overall well-being to give love, share love and therefore, receive love. Feeling loved and being able to share your true feelings usually help to break the vicious cycle of overeating; this cannot be achieved until a person is ready to eliminate the cause for the overeating and breaks the vicious cycle once and for all. A person might not be able to balance their biochemistry through changing eating habits alone. It is of utmost importance for overweight people to be in a loving, harmonious and nurturing relationship.

This relationship occurs when two people are able to learn how to love each other unconditionally and grow spiritually. In such a relationship two souls and two bodies become one, one with all that is. The book *Twin Souls* is recommended to read more about soul growth. This book inspired me to write a screenplay entitled, "*Twin Soul Love.*"

The natural approach to weight loss and healing does not claim to be a substitute for a physician's care, nor does it advocate specific solutions to an individuals problems. Data on health and nutrition are subject to change, as scientists learn more. The living body is a complicated mechanism, and each of us is unique.

I hope you may find the following information useful in leading you to a better way of life.

CONTENTS

Chapter 1

GROWING UP HOLISTICALLY

I was born and raised in Frankfurt, Germany. During my childhood years my mother used homeopathic remedies to help me when I was ill. Homeopathic remedies, usually in the form of plants or minerals, help the body to heal through gentle stimulation. Homeopathy originated in Germany and from there spread throughout Europe.

For 200 years Homeopathy was used in Europe as a safe and gentle tool to restore health with non-toxic remedies. It is the ideal tool for sick children and works on all bodies especially the energy body by removing blockages, therefore, restoring the free flow of energy. The principle of Homeopathy is based on the Law of Similars – "*Like Cures Like.*"

In Germany there are two kinds of pharmacies: One is the Allopathic pharmacy, which generally fills medical doctor's prescription; the other is the Homeopathic pharmacy, which fills prescriptions given by a holistic medical doctor. A person might find Homeopathic and Allopathic pharmacies as well as doctors working on the same premises to help fulfill each person's individual needs.

I personally appreciated such a unique setup. People were given the freedom to choose which way they wanted to restore their health. During my adult years I developed Irritable Bowel Syndrome (IBS), which made it necessary to eliminate whole grains. At that time I could not understand that whole grains could be devastating to some people's health. But by considering blood type, one has the answer. Later on I studied different healing modalities and engaged in more research on blood types.

Giving Birth

In 1972 during my seventh month of pregnancy I was hospitalized with chickenpox. This condition can be deadly to mother and child.

I chose to give birth at a small private hospital run by holistic-oriented doctors. When I fell ill with the chicken pox virus, I decided to go to the same hospital for treatment. If any complications were to arise, the baby could be delivered and treated holistically. There are, however, always exceptions to the rule.

Six weeks later I went into premature labor. The doctor told me that there was no time for the natural birth process. The baby was in danger, and delivery by Caesarian section was required to save the baby's life.

After I came out of the operating room, I was told my baby boy Peter weighed 5 pounds. I could neither hold nor breast-feed him, since he was in critical condition. He was born with meningitis as the chickenpox virus had affected his brain and caused inflammation of the meninges (membranes covering the brain and spinal cord). To stabilize his condition, it was necessary to place Peter in an incubator. The doctor told me there was little they could do except administer antibiotics and anti-seizure medication. They would observe him for a two-to-three month period, as his survival chances were poor. All I could do was visit him daily and look at him through the glass window of the nursery. I felt helpless at that point.

I was devastated upon learning about my son's critical condition. I remember the news like it was yesterday. The doctors were uncertain about Peter's recovery, but I knew in my heart that God could heal him. I started to pray from the bottom of my heart. '*My Father, if it is in accordance with Thy will, please heal Peter. In return, I promise to devote the rest of my life towards helping others to the best of my ability.* "

After three months the doctors released Peter from the hospital, as they could do no more for him. The doctors believed, however, that being born with an **O** blood type gave him the fighting spirit. Peter fought for his life "*like a bear*." In case he survived I should prepare myself for the worst: mental retardation, or living life as a "*zombie*."

I believe God's love and knowing how to apply homeopathic remedies helped Peter to totally recover. At the same time I added small amounts of organic carrot alternating with apple, orange and pear juice, to his formula; this provided him with an excellent source of natural vitamins and minerals to strengthen his immune system. Every evening I applied a small amount of fresh garlic (nature's own antibiotic) to the soles of his feet. I especially included him in my daily prayer. The improvement was slow but steady. After more than a year of medical examinations and many tests the doctors finally agreed that Peter was seizure-free with no traces of brain damage or mental retardation. His general development was delayed during the first two years of his life. The doctors called his recovery a "*miracle*," but I knew in my heart that my prayers had been answered.

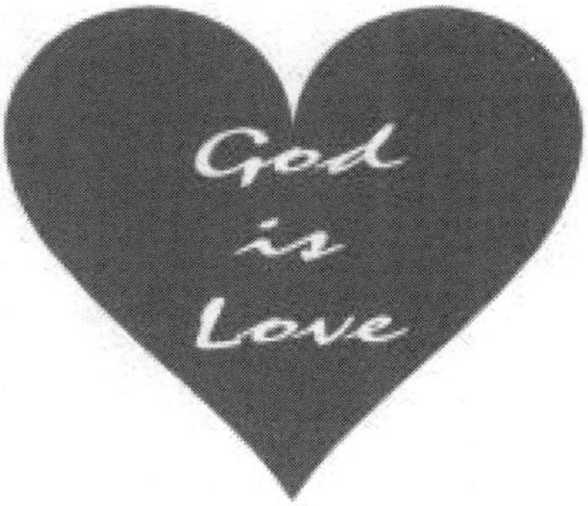

I believe that God uses people every single day to perform miracles through them. After my son's recovery I remembered that I had promised God to help others. I chose to take up the study of holistic health on a full-time basis. I have learned over the years never to ask the question, "*Why me*?" Years from now one will clearly see and understand that the misery and heartaches were needed in order to change one's life for the better.

Never doubt God's intent for miseries and heartaches to be "*blessings in disguise.*" They are life experiences that teach a person compassion for others and to learn how to love unconditionally.

Holistic Health Studies

During my holistic health studies I asked my teachers why they were in favor of vegetarianism. Their reply was that they had tried it and "*it worked.*"

Out of curiosity I asked my teachers if they knew their blood type. Some knew, and not to my surprise the majority were Type **A** and **AB**. These blood types were good candidates for vegetarianism; this explained why they were convinced that everybody could live on a vegetarian diet.

Hippocrates, a holistic medical doctor who lived in 400 B.C., stated; "*Let your food be your medicine and your medicine be your food.*"

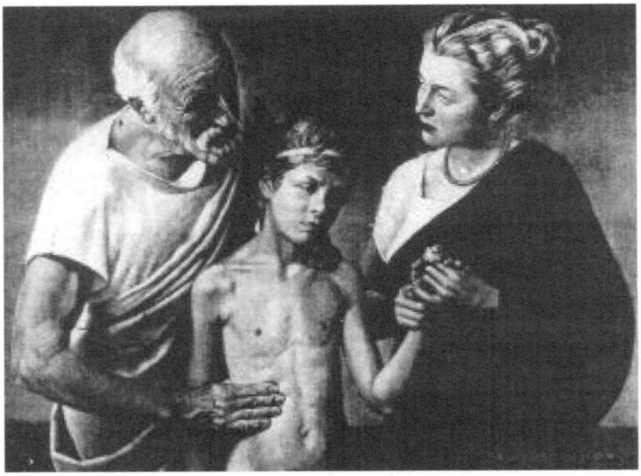

If healthy foods such as whole grains should be your medicine, then why is it possible that such healthy foods could make one sick? The answers I received were unsatisfactory to me.

Later on I came to the conclusion that my health problems were related to my blood type.

I began to relate people's blood types to certain illnesses (page 71).

Now, almost thirty years later, I am able to answer all of my questions by referring to blood types and an individual's unique nutritional needs.

What Are Blood Types?

The Nutrition and Health Encyclopedia defines Blood Types or Groups as **O, A, B, AB** (***AB** being a combination of **A** and **B***). This system of typing is used to prevent incompatible blood transfusion, which can cause serious reactions and sometimes death.

Two blood types are said to be incompatible when the plasma or serum of one blood causes clumping of the cells of the other. Two blood types are said to be compatible and safe for transfusion, if the cells of each can be suspended in the plasma or serum of the other without clumping.

The blood Type **A, B, AB** or **O** is determined by the presence of different mucopolysaccharides (*a substance between collagen fibers*) on the membrane surface of red blood cells. Red blood cells in Type **A** blood are clumped (*agglutinated*) by anti-A serum cells and Type **B** blood are clumped by anti-**B** serum. Type **AB** blood cells are clumped by both serums and Type **O** blood is not clumped by either serum.

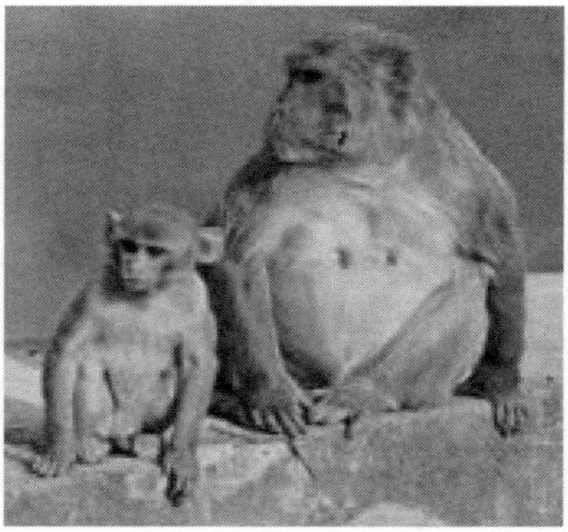

The Rhesus factor (*indicating positive or negative blood*) is named after the Rhesus monkey, a laboratory animal in which this factor was first discovered. The Rhesus factor must be considered, in addition to blood grouping and cross matching for compatibility. The Rh factor is also carried in red blood cells and is found in about 85% of all individuals. These individuals are said to be Rh-positive. As a general rule, the Rh-negative blood can be given to any Rh negative individual.

Type **O** is referred to as *"universal donor"* blood; a term that implies that it can be safely given to any recipient considering the Rh factor. Type **AB** is referred to as *"universal recipient"* blood, considering the Rh factor.

Being an O blood Type, I have always questioned why 15% of the population do not have the Rh factor and are therefore classified as Rh-negative.

After I engaged in religious studies, such as studying the Bible and other Holy Scriptures, as well as reading more books on anthropology (the study of human differences, cultural and biological), I believe I found the answer to my question.

It is stated on several occasions in the Bible (*Genesis 6:1*) "*When men began to increase in number on the earth and daughters were born to them, the sons of God saw that the daughters of men were beautiful, and they married any of them they chose..." With the Nefilim (those whose descendants were on the earth in those days and also afterwards) the sons of God went to the daughters of men and had children by them; they were the heroes of old, men of renown.*" And in Genesis 6:2: "*When the Gods came down from Heaven and mingled with the daughters of men...*"

I believe the interbreeding of the Gods with the daughters of men might not have only changed the Rh factor, it might have also added three more blood types to the one we knew the oldest blood type known to man being Type **O**, the blood type of our ancestors.

Who Are the Gods?

One wonders who are the Gods? In *Eat Right For Your Type*, Peter D'Adamo mentions (page 123) that Great Britain's, Queen Elizabeth II is a Type **O,** as is her son Charles, the Prince of Wales.

In *The Biggest Secret* (page 19), David Icke, an English journalist, agrees with Dr. Arthur David Horn that on the weight of evidence and from his own experience, he is now convinced that humanity was seeded by extraterrestrials and that a *reptilian race* has controlled the planet for thousands of years and continues to do so today. When reading the total of five hundred pages, one will most certainly know what the connection between Great Britain's Queen Elizabeth II, a Type **O** negative, and the reptilian race, considering that the Real Type **O** is the only blood type made to eat and digest meat.

I came to the conclusion that the Rh-positive people are of terra origin and the Rh-negative people are of extraterrestrial origin, the results of the interbreeding.

As Gandhi said it so aptly, *"Even if you are in a minority of one, the truth is still the truth."* Recommended reading on our extraterrestrial origin:

The Old Testament
Humanity's Extraterrestrial Origins
The Biggest Secret
Star Gods, Clone Masters of the Universe
On our terra origin:
Blood relations, Blood Groups and Anthropology

Chapter 2

DR. LANDSTEINER

In 1900 the great Austrian pathologist Dr. Landsteiner was the first to discover that people do not all belong to the same blood group. He received the *Nobel Prize* for his great contribution in 1930.

Dr. Landsteiner demonstrated that red blood cells in some individuals produced a substance called anti-body. He made this discovery by mixing different individuals' blood together. He also proved that humans could be classified into four groups on the basis of these naturally occurring antibodies.

The renowned Max Planck Institute, The Center for Nutritional Research, is located in Frankfurt, Germany. A few years ago they moved their headquarters to Berlin, Germany. The Max Planck Institute did major research on blood type varieties by collecting scientific data during World War 1 (1914 - 1918) on wounded soldiers.

These researchers came to the conclusion that one medication used on four various blood types produced four different results. This study answered my question of whether a person's unique biochemical make-up could determine their nutritional needs including supplemental or medicinal needs.

Chapter 3

NON-VEGETARIANS VS. VEGETARIANS

Research indicates that the North American population represents:

Type **O** blood group approximately 44%

Type **B** blood group approximately 10%

I refer to these types as the meat and fish-eating blood groups or simply as non-vegetarians.

Type **A** blood group approximately 42%

Type **AB** blood group approximately 4%

I refer to these types as the vegetable eating blood group or vegetarians.

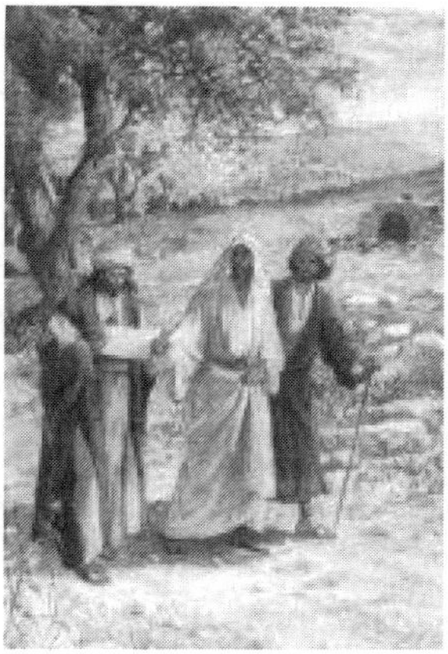

It is believed that during Biblical times, people lived solely off whatever the Earth had to offer. Some lived strictly off the land, farming or hunting, while others were drawn to the sea for their food supply.

Defining Metabolism

Metabolism is defined as the process by which foods are transformed into basic elements (*nutrients*), which can be used by the body for energy, growth and maintenance of good health. To maintain a person's ideal weight, it is advisable to consume foods, which are compatible with their blood type; otherwise, the individual may experience weight gain.

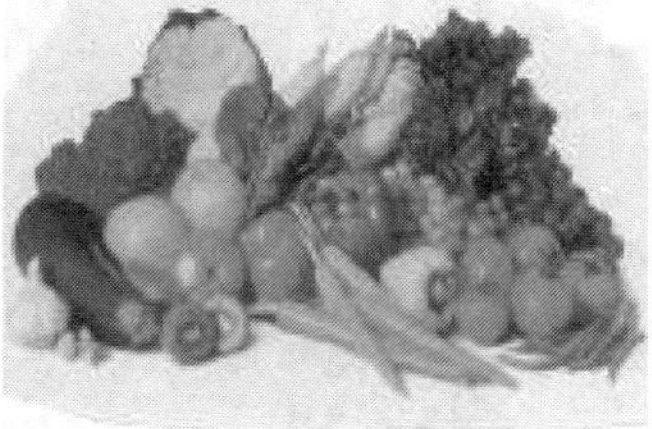

All food should be consumed in its natural state with little or no processing by eliminating all refined (and especially genetically altered) foods.

The reason for the above advice is that uncooked foods contain all the enzymes needed by the body to properly digest. The cooking and refining process destroy enzymes, and thus, one eats more or less "*dead food*."

Are Supplements Needed?

What supplements should one take to stay healthy and prolong life? My answer depends on a person's blood Type (including parents blood types) and the spiritual awareness, as well as the level of stress on a daily basis.

I believe that if a person eats natural unprocessed and wholesome foods and has no particular health problem, one is able to derive nutrients. This belief applies especially to Types **A** and **AB**. Supplements may not be required at all by Types **A** and **AB.** A person may desire to supplement such as blue green algae, chlorella, spirulina and naturally grown vitamins and minerals ("*Pure Synergy*", page 119). An added supplement is homeostatic soil organisms (HSO), which are further discussed in this chapter. Types **A** and **AB** also benefit from herbal combination formulas, and homeopathic plant-based remedies, avoiding glandular extracts.

Homeopathic remedies should be taken in pellet form avoiding the alcohol-based extracts. All synthetic unnatural supplements should be avoided; these may cause more harm than good and may be deposited in a person's body when taken over prolonged periods.

Multivitamins should be taken on a short-term basis. I am not in favor of multivitamins and minerals. However, to illustrate this point, consider the following example: a person might only require three nutrients out of ten and the rest may be stored in the liver as toxins.

Types **A, AB** and **B** who engage in smoking and drinking need to supplement their diet according to their type. This group includes people who have taken antibiotics and others who eat refined processed foods on a regular basis.

Probiotics

In general there are two supplements I recommend taking no matter what blood type.

The first supplement is called "*Probiotics,*" known as the "*friendly intestinal bacteria.*" This supplement maintains healthy intestinal flora necessary for proper digestion and assimilation of food. *Probiotics* include *Lactobacillus acidophilus*, *bifidus*, *faecicum*, *rhamnosus* and others. *Lactobacillus acidophilus* can reduce high cholesterol levels and is capable of destroying the yeast known as *candida albicans*. *Bifidus* is the first bacteria given to babies through mother's milk, which keeps the baby's intestine healthy. *Faecicum* is mainly used to reverse diarrhea. All of these *probiotics* are indigenous to the human lower intestinal tract. *Rhamnosus* was discovered more recently and helps in protein digestion and preventing harmful bacteria from attaching to the intestinal walls.

I usually recommend dairy-free *probiotics* for Types **A** and **AB**, preferably the one cultured on apple pectin and nothing else added, the kind without the fructo oligosaccarides (FOS). *Acidophilus*, *bifidus faecicum* and *rhamnosus* cultured on lactose or goat's milk are recommended for Types **O** and **B**. One capsule usually consists of approximately 5 to 10 billion of friendly bacteria and should be taken without FOS. The reason for this is that FOS is added most often to *probiotics* to feed the friendly bacteria. However, at the same time, it feeds the pathogenic (harmful) bacteria and can exacerbate one's health problem, especially if you suffer from Candidiasis (yeast infection, page 74) or any other bacterial or viral infection.

Probiotics are available at most health food stores. Be sure to check the label. The ideal is *Lactobacillus acidophilus*, by itself or in combination with *bifidus*. You might find *acidophilus* in conjunction with *bulgaricus*, *faecicum* or *rhamnosus*. All need to be kept in the refrigerator to keep the bacteria alive and active.

Bifidus and *acidophilus* are beneficial for children experiencing either diarrhea or the flu. *Probiotics* are harmless and have no side effects. I even feed *probiotics* to my pets to keep them healthy. Children might prefer taking the *acidophilus* and/or *bifidus* as liquid (Bio-K) or powder (*Organika and Natural Factors*) added to their juice.

Homeostatic Soil Organisms (HSO)

Homeostatic Soil Organisms (HSO) are other beneficial bacteria capable of balancing the acid/alkaline pH (potential hydrogen) while at the same time ridding the intestinal tract of putrefaction and pathogenic (harmful) organisms. William C. Bryce, M.D., Ph.D., who wrote a research paper on soil organisms, states that, *"As HSO destroy molds, yeast, fungus and viruses in the soil of the organic garden, they perform the same with pathological organisms in the gut, greatly augmenting the body's immune system*."

Types **A** and **AB** seem to respond best to HSO due to being the descendants of the farmers. HSO can be taken in conjunction with *probiotics* as they usually complement each other. One might try alternating them to see which beneficial bacterium works best; you might also want to test them prior to taking (page 115).

Homeopathy

The second group of supplements is called homeopathic remedies. Homeopathic remedies are not really supplements at all. As previously discussed, homeopathic remedies work on a subtle energy level by restoring balance to the body. Homeopathic remedies can prevent or cure illness by activating the body's inborn healing mechanism.

Homeopathic remedies are capable of removing physical or emotional trauma. They are some of the safest tools known to man, safe enough to give to children and pets.

Considering a person's blood type, the experienced homeopath would avoid administering glandular extract to Types **A** and **AB**, the so-called vegetarians. Types **A** and **AB** will respond better to a remedy derived from plants and minerals.

Homeopathic glandulars would be a fitting choice for Types **O** and **B**. Satisfactory results would occur when considering biochemical individuality.

The question arises, can one really prolong life, prevent illness by living in tune with the body, listening and satisfying all its needs? This idea definitely assures a better quality of life, but as to whether one can prolong life, the best advice is to consider the old saying; "*Prevention is better than cure.*"

Chapter 4

REAL TYPE "O" SUPPLEMENTS

The Real Type **O** has a high-energy body and often seems to be involved in stressful situations. This type often seems to be living life on the edge, unable to live a sedentary life and needs to be physically active, needing challenges on a daily basis. The Real Type **O** seeks executive, nerve-racking positions. This is in contrast to the Type **A** who prefers a sedentary life.

In general, the Real Type **O** needs to supplement with antioxidants, especially if smoking cigarettes or drinking alcohol.

My husband is a real Type **O** and a smoker; I supplement his diet with the following:

Supplement	Dosage	Potency
Super halibut liver oil (A)	1 gel caps	10.000 iu
Super halibut liver oil (D)		400 iu
Beta-carotene	1 capsule	25.000 iu
B complex	1 capsule	50 mg
Ester C with Bioflavonoids	1 capsule	600 mg
Quercetin	1 capsule	600 mg
Natural Vitamin E	1 capsule	400 iu
Selenium oxide	1 tablet	50 mcg
Chromium Picolinate	1 tablet	200 mcg
Magnesium oxide	1 tablet	250 mg
Zinc Citrate	1 tablet	50 mg
Co-enzyme Q10	1 capsule	30 mg
Ginkgo biloba	1 capsule	600 mg
Saw palmetto	1 capsule	500 mg
Colostrum	1 capsule	500 mg
Microhydrin	1 capsule	250 mg
Organic Spirulina	3 tablets	1000 mg
Acidophilus (Probiotic)	1 capsule	10 billion

These supplements are taken six days a week, resting on the seventh day. Quantity depends on the stress level and the ability to release stress and relax on a daily basis.

Antioxidants

Why are antioxidants and other supplements beneficial to a Type **O** smoker? To answer this question, let us consider the following:

1.) What are antioxidants?

In general antioxidants are substances such as vitamin A, the B complex, beta-carotene, vitamin C and bioflavonoids, quercetin (another bioflavonoid), natural vitamin E (d tocopherol) plus selenium, grape seed extract and microhydrin. These antioxidants are capable of protecting cells from free radicals damage.

2.) What are free radicals?

Free radicals are highly reactive molecules capable of damaging cells and tissue. Free radical formation increases with stress, including: illness, smoking cigarettes, drinking alcohol and from environmental pollutants. Antioxidants are needed to neutralize the damaging effects of the free radicals on a cellular level.

3.) Vitamins A and D (antioxidants)

Vitamins A and D, derived from fish oil, are recommended for Types **O** or **B**. Vitamin A, derived from lemongrass, as well as beta-carotene, is recommended for Types **A** and **AB**.

The fish oil variety can be stored in the body and need not be replenished every day, especially when taken in larger doses than normally required. I am not in favor of taking more than 5,000 to 10,000 iu a day.

Vitamin A keeps the outer layer of the tissues and organs healthy. In a smoker Vitamin A prevents damage to the respiratory system.

Vitamin A is capable of fighting infections and viral invasion in conjunction with vitamin C. Vitamin A also prevents shrinkage of the thymus gland and works best in conjunction with beta-carotene.

4.) Beta-carotene (antioxidant)

Beta-carotene is a precursor of vitamin A, also known as pro-vitamin A. They work in conjunction, enhancing each other's antioxidant properties. Some people, especially diabetics, are unable to convert beta-carotene into vitamin A; which could possibly be stored in the liver and lead to toxicity.

5.) B complex (antioxidant)

The B complex consists of water-soluble vitamins, that work together as co-enzymes. They are needed for proper carbohydrate, protein and fat metabolism. The complex is also needed for cell reproduction and a healthy nervous system.

6.) Vitamin C (antioxidant)

Vitamin C is a weak acid, it is capable of killing bacteria, fungi and parasites, therefore, it is useful with all kinds of infections. Vitamin C also strengthens tissues and works synergistically with other vitamins to enhance their properties. Most humans cannot obtain vitamin C from food alone, especially Types **O** and **B**. These blood types need to supplement. Vitamin C comes in many different forms.

I usually recommend the buffered kind, especially when a person has stomach problems. The form of Ester C is supposed to be the most effective vitamin C. Some vegetarians, however, might prefer the naturally derived rosehip variety. Vitamin C's absorption is enhanced when taken along with bioflavonoids derived from lemon, orange and/or grapefruit.

7.) Bioflavonoids (antioxidant)

Bioflavonoids are a group of water soluble nutrients derived mostly form orange, lemon and grapefruit; they are similar to the action of vitamin C and are capable of strengthening capillaries and reducing inflammation. These nutrients are also known for their anti-cancer and anti-viral properties. Bioflavonoids work best in conjunction with vitamin C.

8.) Quercetin (antioxidant)

Quercetin is the most potent of the bioflavonoids, which enhance vitamin C activity.

9.) Vitamin E (antioxidant)

Vitamin E protects the body from harmful pollutants and other nutrients from being damaged by free radicals. Vitamin E is needed to heal injured tissue and to prevent scarring.

10.) Selenium oxide (antioxidant)

Selenium works in conjunction with vitamin E to fight free radical damage. Selenium binds to toxic metals and keeps them from being absorbed.

11.) Chromium Picolinate

Chromium is best known as the blood-sugar stabilizer. Diabetics and hypoglycemics especially need it. A deficiency of chromium will be seen in overweight people, as well as in people who live on a refined carbohydrate diet. Chromium keeps arteries healthy in conjunction with other minerals.

12.) Magnesium oxide

Magnesium and calcium work synergistically. One usually gets plenty of calcium but not enough magnesium when consuming large amounts of dairy products.

Calcium constricts muscles and magnesium relaxes muscles. Magnesium is a natural potent immune nutrient.

13.) Zinc Citrate

Zinc is an important trace mineral. Its properties are enhanced when taken with vitamin A, as the two work synergistically. It is now commonly accepted that zinc is required in older men to keep the prostate healthy. Zinc is also needed for proper carbohydrate digestion. Zinc prevents arteriosclerosis and speeds up wound healing.

14.) Co-enzyme Q10

Co-enzyme Q10 is classified as an essential nutrient needed in the production of energy within the cell. This nutrient is capable of preventing arteriosclerosis and heart disease and works synergistically with vitamin E.

15.) Ginkgo biloba (antioxidant)

The herb ginkgo is also classified as an antioxidant. It is known to slow formation of free radicals and acts as a vasodilating agent. It helps cerebral and vascular conditions by widening blood vessels, thus increasing circulation, and is also used to prevent premature aging.

16.) Saw palmetto

The herb saw palmetto as a tissue builder and aids in keeping the respiratory system and prostate healthy.

17.) Colostrum

Taken from veterinary-certified, healthy pesticide and hormone-free cows, colostrum is the first food all mammals receive from their mother. Colostrum is responsible for giving the newborn excellent nutrition, thus enhancing immune function and therefore preventing disease. As we all know, maintaining a healthy immune system is essential for optimum health.

18.) Microhydrin (silica, potassium carbonate and magnesium sulfate antioxidant)

Microhydrin provides a high concentration of negative hydrogen ions, encased in micro clusters that produce an antioxidant effect. Microhydrin is 2,000 times stronger than vitamin C; it removes toxins from inside the cell and increases absorption of other nutrients to 100%.

19.) Organic Spirulina (a green food supplement)

Organic Spirulina contains mixed carotenoids and antioxidants as well as phytonutrients, contains essential fatty acids and is high in B12 and iron.

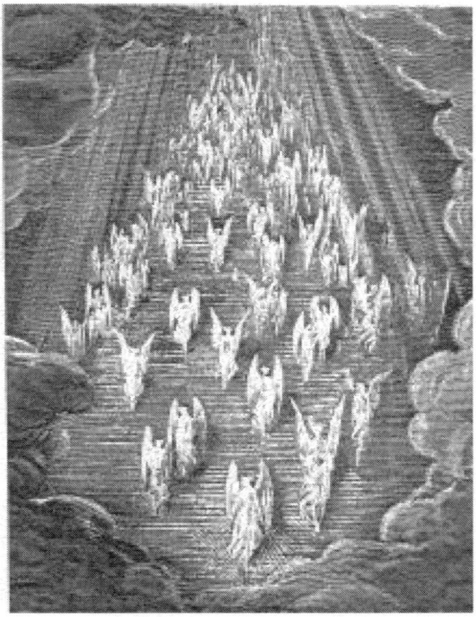

The previously mentioned supplements are taken by my husband to minimize free radical damage to his cells and tissue to keep his respiratory system free from smoke-inhalation damage. It would be much better to eliminate his smoking habit, instead of trying to compensate by taking supplements. However, I have been told many times that it is much easier to take supplements than it is to change his life style. I totally agree. However, I believe it is a person's duty to keep the physical body (the temple of God) healthy by eating natural unprocessed foods (preferably organically grown) in accordance with nature's law. Living a loving harmonious life and practicing stress release through daily exercise, according to your blood type, helps to reduce stress.

Entertaining positive thoughts only keeps the mental body functioning properly. Keeping your emotions calm and under control can help a great deal in preserving your health.

Practicing daily communications (prayer) with the Heavenly Father, Earthly Mother, their Archangels and Angels, keeps your spiritual body well-nourished and therefore, healthy. It is important to keep in mind at all times that "*God's love heals all.*"

Pasteurized and Homogenized Milk vs. Non-pasteurized and Non-homogenized Milk

The pasteurization of milk destroys all enzymes and heat-labile nutrients. This process changes the chemical structures of proteins and fats in the milk and makes milk hard to digest. Heat-processed milk and cheese can create allergies in sensitive people, such as Types **A** and **AB**. Most of the time, however, these allergies are not related to the pasteurization of the milk.

Some consumers are so brainwashed that they believe the media hype that non-pasteurized (raw) milk is dangerous to your health. Parents have the responsibility to provide their children with wholesome foods, making sure they provide all the nutrients needed for growth and well-being. Pasteurized milk is not a good choice. If non-pasteurized, organic milk is used to make yogurt and cheese, then all the enzymes needed for digestion are still alive, and dairy products are more easily digested.

However, if one were unable to obtain non-pasteurized (raw) milk the other alternative would be to consume yogurt instead of drinking milk. By adding *lactobacillus acidophilus* to the pasteurized milk, the dead milk is brought back to life. Keep in mind that yogurt is more easily digested than drinking milk. If one cannot get used to the taste of yogurt, adding 1-2 tbsp. of fresh lemon juice to a glass of milk (stir with a plastic spoon) makes the milk curdle and therefore, easier to digest, adding vitamin C and potassium as well.

On the other hand, you can always consider owning your own cow to provide your own organic raw milk.

I know what the so-called experts answer would be: Pasteurization is needed to destroy all pathogenic (harmful) bacteria in the milk, which might otherwise cause a health problem.

My response to this statement is cows eating grass that has not been chemically treated with pesticides produce organic milk. The cow's meal is also supplemented with organically grown feed, grown without chemicals such as antibiotics, pesticides, insecticides currently used to increase milk production. It is these additives that cause allergic reactions in sensitive people. A veterinarian checks organic cows on a monthly basis to insure that they are healthy. Therefore, the risk of becoming sick by ingesting organic milk is eliminated.

Homogenization of milk is a process, which emulsifies the fats in the milk. Is homogenization of milk better than pasteurization? Kurt Oster's research indicates that during the homogenization process xanthine oxidase (XO) found in the milk fat is released. XO can enter the bloodstream, endangering a person's health by leaving scars on arterial walls.

The answer to the above would be to commercialize and promote non-pasteurized milk from healthy cows, which graze on unsprayed grass and are organically fed.

To improve the digestion of milk, you can take digestive enzymes or the enzyme lactase. Lactase is needed to digest the lactose in milk; this may help but is not a solution, simply a crutch. The solution is raw foods derived from fruits, vegetables, and plants. Using non-pasteurized milk products supplies the body with enzymes and nutrients needed for proper digestion.

Another frequently asked question is: How much protein is needed for the overall well-being of Types **A** and **AB** in comparison to Types **O** and **B**?

As stated previously, research indicates that Types **A** and **AB** are most suitable for an all-vegetarian/fruit diet. Their need for protein is usually low, approximately 30 grams. This lack of protein can be easily obtained by adding soya products, legumes, nuts, seeds and grains to their vegetable and fruit diet. Sprouted grains are preferred due to being less acidic.

Most Type **A** and **AB** are unable to digest or assimilate proteins of animal origin except some plain *acidophilus* yogurt (preferably homemade). In general, they do well on a so-called high-complex (unrefined) carbohydrate, low-protein diet. On the other hand, Types **O** and **B** do not do well on an all-vegetarian diet, due to their hunter and fisher origins.

Types **O** might have difficulties digesting soya or whole-grain products. Even legumes and nuts might cause a problem. Types **O** and **B** have higher protein requirements, approximately 60 grams. They might need to add some animal protein; such as meat, fish, eggs, organic non-pasteurized (raw) cheese and yogurt to their vegetable and fruit diet.

In general, Types **O** and **B** do well on a so-called high-protein low-carbohydrate diet. However, high protein intake does not mean one has to overeat. Everything consumed should be in accordance to the bodily needs and no one can tell someone else how much that will be. Only through listening to the body will you know what quantity of foods is required to well sustain the body. Always remember biochemical uniqueness (food testing is recommended, page 115).

When Type **O** does eliminate all meat and convert to vegetarianism, they are sometimes afraid of not getting enough protein. But following the above example there is no reason for concern. According to the Max Planck Institute one usually consumes too much protein to begin with. This excess protein is then stored in the body, where it is able to cause all kinds of health problems (page 71).

Readers may not be familiar with the fact that almost everything they eat is loaded with protein. Fruit supplies the same percentage of complete protein as mother's milk. In general, when proteins from animal or even vegetable sources are eaten in excess, the subtle energy body slows down and becomes almost non-existent.

When counting carbohydrates, it is advisable to reduce fruit intake to a minimum, while substituting fruit with vegetables. The same advice applies when bothered by recurring Candidiasis (yeast infection, page 74)

Protein from Eggs?

In considering becoming a vegetarian, a frequently asked question is: Is it all right to become lacto-ova vegetarian, including eggs and dairy products?

Personally, I feel that adding some dairy to the diet is acceptable. Eating eggs, however, is totally up to that person's spiritual belief. I am not in favor of eggs as I believe to eat eggs is to kill another being.

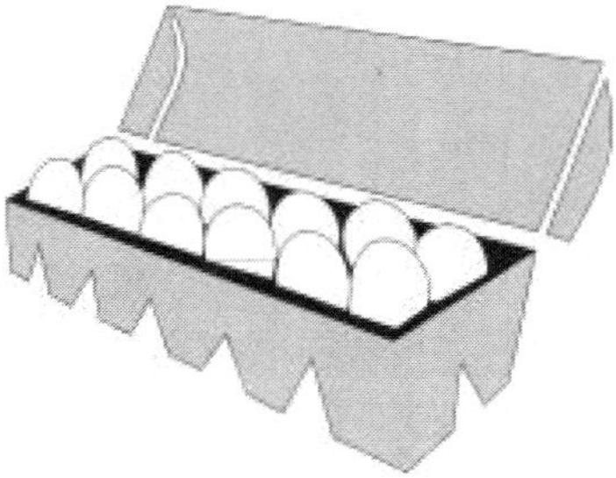

Usually, the answer is that eating unfertilized eggs would not be killing; however, that is only partially correct. An egg remains unfertilized only because the appropriate circumstance for its fertilization has been withheld. Therefore, the egg cannot complete its natural purpose of developing into a chicken. Even though this development has not occurred, it still contains the innate (inborn) life force needed for such development.

As mentioned above, it is advisable to eat all foods in their natural state. Meat and fish should be eaten grilled, without batter. However, there is always the exception to the rule. It is important to learn to listen to the body and its needs; this requires raising your consciousness through prayer.

Through studying and applying the blood type concept to myself, I was able to understand my own biochemical uniqueness. I am Type **O** negative. Since I am a combination of Type **O** and **B**, I am not as tough as a 100% Type **O**. In actuality, I have been very sensitive my whole life. I especially noticed the difference between my husband, a real Type **O**, and myself. My husband seems to get away with everything in contrast to me.

If I were to try to live his life, I would not survive a single day. Thus, it is of utmost importance to know one's parent's blood types. Knowing this can be a difficult task, especially if they no longer walk on this earth. Fortunately, during my blood type studies my mother was still around for me to question. I just wanted to know if I am a real Type **O** or a combination of a Type **O** and another blood type. I am a Type **O** negative on my mother's side but not on my father's side. My father was Type **B** negative; therefore, I am a combination of the two. I classify myself as a Type **OB** negative.

Once I knew my father's blood type, I was able to answer my questions. For instance, in the past I never liked meat, but eating a little fish once in a while felt all right to me.

Chapter 5

THE ESSENE GOSPEL OF PEACE

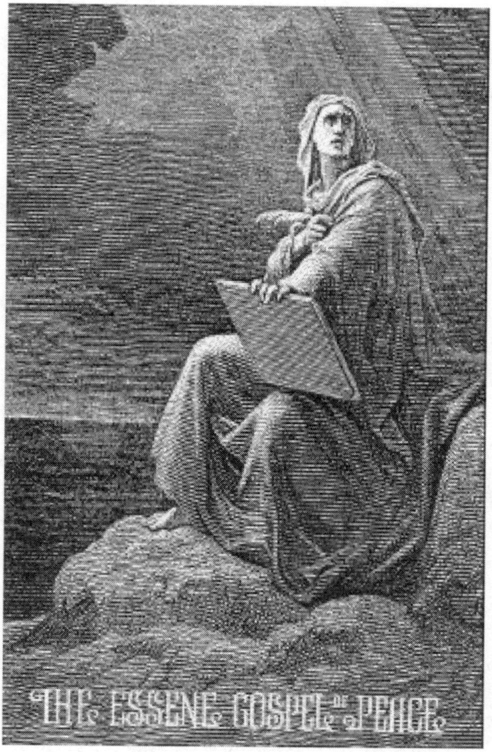

Once I studied various Holy books and started living a more harmonious life through prayer and meditation, I was able to raise my vibration frequency of my body to a level where animal meat was no longer needed to sustain my body. A few years ago, I was given a book called: *The Essene Gospel of Peace*. This book is believed to contain Jesus' lost teachings in which He states, "What it takes to have a healthy body, mind, and spirit." I lovingly refer to the book as, *Jesus' Little Diet Book*.

Most of humanity is not aware that such a book exists. After I read the book, I knew that I was on the right path. The last few years I have proved to myself that even a Type **O** can become at least a lacto-vegetarian when one desires to do so. It takes time to learn (listen to one's body) how to substitute animal protein such as meat and fish, etc. with non-pasteurized dairy, nuts, seeds, vegetables and fruit in a balanced way (quality and quantity counts). To attain this balance, one needs to keep in mind that we are all spiritual beings on an earthly mission and that we are surrounded by energy. All is energy and energy can be rearranged (page 90).

Edgar Cayce said it well in a book, titled, *There Is a River*, by Thomas Sugrue. The human body is made up of electronic vibrations, with each atom and element of the body, each organ and organism having its electronic unit of vibration necessary for the sustenance of, and equilibrium in, that particular organism.

Each unit, then, being a cell or a unit of life in itself has the capacity to reproduce itself by the first law known as reproduction-division. When a force in any organ or element of the body becomes deficient in its ability to reproduce that equilibrium necessary for the sustenance of physical existence and its reproduction, that portion is deficient in electronic energy. This deficiency may come by injury or disease, be received by external forces, or come from internal forces through lack of eliminations produced in the system or by other agencies to meet its requirements in the body.

Type **O** can change to a certain extent one's biochemistry. However, Type **O** usually never desires to become a fruitarian. This desire is most of the time only achieved by Type **A** and **AB**.

By eating dense foods such as meat, fish, fried eggs, pasteurized dairy products, processed and deep-fried foods, the vibration frequency of the body is lowered.

On the other hand, if one eliminates most of the dense foods, the body begins to vibrate at a higher frequency. Spiritual energy can actually take over by healing and even sustaining the body. If the reader is interested to know more about subtle energies, Gabriel Cousens, M.D. explains these phenomena in detail in *Spiritual Nutrition And The Rainbow Diet*.

When one engages in a spiritual fast, these subtle energies, which surround us, are capable of sustaining the body.

All Holy Scriptures recommend fasting and praying as tools to become one with God. If one seeks healing, it is believed that fasting and praying speed up the healing process.

A fast does not necessarily mean one must eliminate all foods. Fasting actually means to eat less and lighter foods, such as fruit, fruit juice, and/or vegetable juice, while eliminating all solid food for a few days.

A fast also means taking attention off food and concentrating more on God, the Creator. I must admit it took me two years to change my body from a low vibration frequency to a higher vibration frequency.

In my case sometimes the frequency of my body is too high to feel comfortable to live with. This discomfort occurs especially in the summertime, when I am trying to eat just fruits and nothing else. I become easily light-headed. However, adding a little yogurt or soured milk to my fruit helps to balance my vibrations.

You must learn to take in just the right food and amount of food to maintain a balanced body, and this takes time. Keep in mind that you cannot force your body to become a vegetarian. As much as you have prepared yourself physically and mentally you may not really be ready for such a change in eating habits. For example, Type **O** needs lots of time to switch from an all-meat diet to a vegetarian diet. However, I am often told, that after reading *The Essene Gospel of Peace*, you will feel divinely guided, and the transition from an all-meat diet to a vegetarian diet is easier than you thought it would be.

Chapter 6

ACKNOWLEDGING THE ONENESS IN ALL

I refer to the blood type diet as the first step. This first step leads to an ideal weight and a balanced body. If that is all you seek as a goal, then that is all right. The second step I call the path to freedom. This step is more difficult to achieve but possibly depending on your desire and purpose. Besides reducing or eliminating dense foods, you must learn to open your heart and unconditionally love all of God's creation.

There is such a thing as *"Universal laws."* When all laws combined represent the *"One Law,"* this is unity; and man is an inseparable part of it. It is this unity that makes man a co-creator with the Creator, who is supposed to take care of and preserve his creation. To be part of the *"One Law"* includes: To love and honor others and ourselves unconditionally, planet Earth our home and all sentient beings in it through acknowledging their sacredness and our unity. By doing so one is able to love from the heart. By practicing unconditional love towards all kingdoms, one remembers the sixth of the Ten Commandments: "*Thou shall not kill.*"

The book, *The Seat Of The Soul*, is a great tool to align the personality with the all-loving soul. However, if still feeling unable to love unconditionally, one might want to ask the Heavenly Father in prayer to send divine love through you, to all one comes in contact with. And since God is all love, it is easy to do. It is said: "Love transcends all."

No matter into what race we are born, we are all brothers and sisters, all God's children. When away from home on an earthly mission, we are eager to go home again once our mission is fulfilled. Some might fulfill their mission sooner, some later, mostly depending on how much we are able to love from the heart, loving unconditionally.

It might be of interest to know our brother's and sister's blood type and how blood types in general relate to a particular race. In North America, most of Types **A** and **AB** are found in the asian and black races. On the other hand, most Types **O** and **B** are found in the caucasian and native american races.

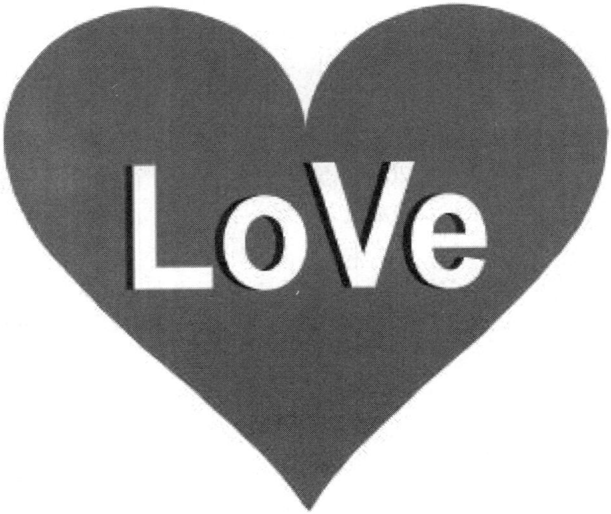

Chapter 7

COMPATIBLE PARTNERS

Today people look for a "soul mate", not knowing that the term soul mate refers to all humans on earth. All humans have a soul and are mates. What they really seek is their "twin soul", which is literally the other half of themselves and is the most compatible partner. There is a big difference between these two types of mates. The book Twin Souls explains the difference and the twin soul connection in detail.

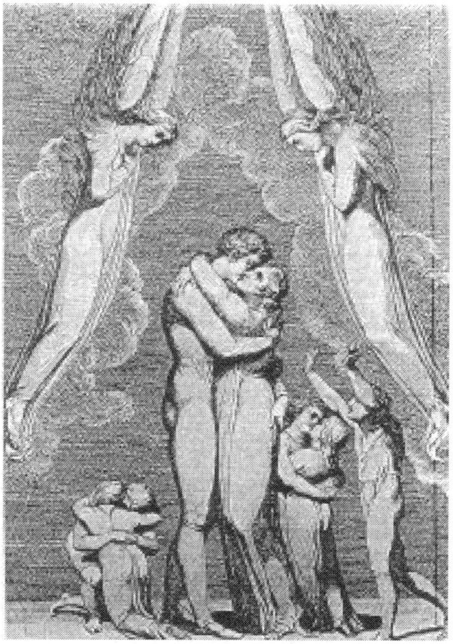

There has to be absolute surety of what one is trying (through prayer) to manifest into life. The movie, *Twin Soul Love*, shows the difference between the different loves and what the real meaning is on a "soul" level.

From my own research, the most compatible physical partner is the one with the same blood type and Rhesus factor, therefore indicating the same origin (terra- or extra-terrestrial.)

The Greek philosopher Pythagoras [598-504 B.C.], the inventor of our current mathematical system, the science of numbers, stated that to know numbers and their significance is to know one's self, leading to knowledge of a "Twin Soul."

Socrates, Aristotle and Plato believed that one's life path is based on numbers. St. Augustine studied numbers for their religious significance. Psychologist Carl Jung believed that a number is quantity as well as meaning. However, please keep in mind that God makes the final decision, because everything happens according to the divine plan.

Chapter 8

PROPER AND CONSCIOUS EATING

It is important to never rush through a meal. When in a hurry, it is better not to eat at all. One should sit quietly with a relaxed body and mind, in order to digest and assimilate food properly, thanking God for one's daily food and blessing it.

If one wants to lose weight it is recommended to chew your food slowly, thus satisfying the hunger feeling without having to overeat. It is advisable to eat proteins such as meat, fish, eggs, cheese, nuts, seeds and legumes first, followed by vegetables and salad. The reason for this is that hydrochloric acid, needed to digest proteins, is released at the beginning of one's meal and slows down toward the end.

Most restaurants serve salad first and about 15 to 20 minutes later the main course (protein) is served. This method of serving impairs protein digestion. Salad and vegetables do not need hydrochloric acid to be digested, but protein does. Most of the time, making this small adjustment can help prevent indigestion.

It is easier to eat protein first when dining at buffet restaurants, because you are able to choose the foods you want to eat first. On the other hand, I do not recommend buffet restaurants, because they present a great temptation to overeat. Personally, I am not in favor of restaurant-prepared foods. One never knows what one is getting, especially nowadays where genetically altered foods are served as well!

It is advisable to eat the main protein meal at noon. After 3:00 pm the hydrochloric acid production in the stomach, needed for protein digestion, slows down. Evening meals should consist mainly of starches, or starch less vegetables depending on one's blood type. For improved digestion vegetables and salads with little or no protein are best.

If one likes to drink with meals, drinks are best served at room temperature. Drinks too hot or too cold can also impair proper digestion. If proteins were taken at dinner time, it would be advisable to eat the protein meal no later than 7:00 p.m. Proteins such as red meat, nuts, and seeds are all stimulants, as much as coffee and tea, as are herbal teas such as green and peppermint tea. With any of these drinks at or after dinner, you might have difficulty falling asleep.

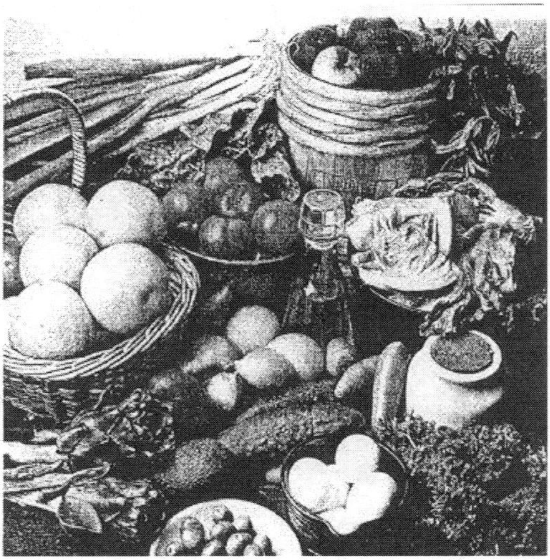

Most nutritionists recommend eating a main protein meal for lunch and starches and salads for dinner (preferably according to blood type and using food testing, (page 115).

Ideal Living Conditions

As mentioned earlier, I was born and raised in the major business city of Frankfurt, Germany. Being born an only child into a family in the hotel and restaurant business, it was expected that I would take over the business once I had completed Hotel and Restaurant Management School. I managed the hotel and restaurant for a few years, until my son Peter was born. As you know by now, it was for this reason that I discontinued my profession to take up the study of holistic health on a full-time basis.

During the last 27 years my family and I have lived in many different countries, searching for the ideal spot to raise a family while at the same time, being able to reconnect with nature. We believe we have finally found the perfect spot. We bought a little fruit farm in the Niagara Region of Ontario, Canada, and no longer needed a major city to call home.

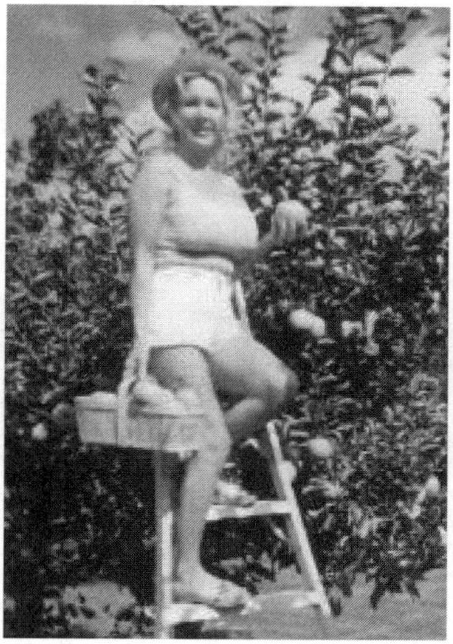

We converted the fruit farm into an all-organic fruit farm, viewing the farm work as a hobby. I believe the ideal living condition is provided by living on a piece of land in the country away from the hustle and bustle of a major city. This kind of location is especially good when seeking peace of mind after a hectic day at the office. Surrounding oneself with trees has a tremendous calming and balancing effect on the whole body. Walking through, or working with trees, is the most natural stress release there is, allowing us to connect with Mother Nature.

I consider farm work and gardening a pleasure, to work with nature. In the summertime I really enjoy being able to pick my own fruit for lunch and dinner.

I know that our fruit is nutritious, as it is free of herbicides, pesticides and is not genetically altered. Please remember that Type **O** does best when fruit is eaten in moderation. It gives me great satisfaction in life to look after mother earth the way it was meant to be cared for.

Chapter 9

My Diet – My Lifestyle

I usually wake up with the birds. The first hour I engage in bathing and dressing myself. The second hour is devoted to God in prayer and meditation, defining meditation; listening to God's answer to my prayers. Then I am ready for the challenges of the day.

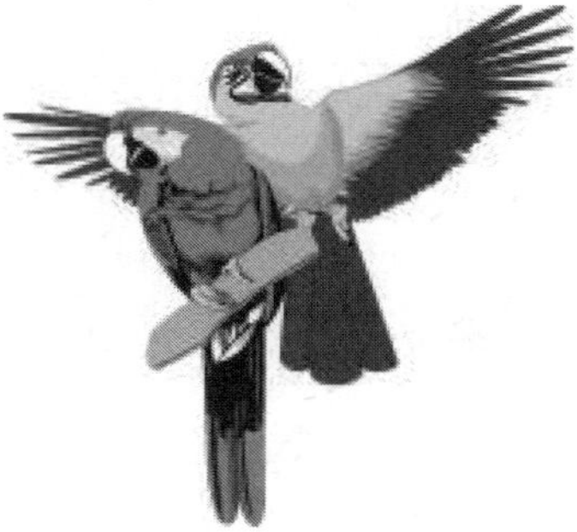

I do not eat or drink anything until noon, my main protein meal consisting of:

- 75 grams organic, raw, mild cheddar cheese
- 50 grams of pecans or walnuts
- 1 papaya (for protein digestion)

Glass of organic soured (lemon) milk with 1 tbsp. organic milled flaxseeds, sesame seeds and hemp seeds (nuts) and 1 tbsp. organic spirulina added.

1 piece of seasonal fruit.

- Bowl of navy beans topped with hummus (page 105)
- 1/2 jar of homemade yogurt.
- 1 small apple or pear.

I take the following supplements with a 12-oz glass of Vittel water, at room temperature, (the only bottled water I tolerate): 500 mg. magnesium oxide (a natural alkalizer, relaxant and powerful immune nutrient), 1000 mg of natural B12 with folic, 100 mcg, sublingually (the only way to take B12 for it to be absorbed properly) or by injection. I seem to need B12 mostly in wintertime, due to spending less time in the sunshine. Sunshine is known to invigorate the body, the same feeling one gets when taking B12.

If in need of a pick-me-up in the afternoon, B12 can do that more naturally and safer than any coffee or alcohol. Some Type **O**'s might need to supplement extra B12 with folic acid, especially when converting from an all-meat diet to a vegetarian diet. Red meat is loaded with B12, but sometimes Type **O**'s might need extra B12, more than obtained from vegetables and spirulina.

I also take 800 iu of natural vitamin E (mixed tocopherol). However, I do not take it orally, I apply 800 iu of natural vitamin E plus a little flax mixed with hemp seed, evening primrose and *rosa mosqueta* oil to my face at night. This moisturizer is known to erase fine lines and is worthwhile trying. Anything applied to the skin is immediately absorbed into the body; that is why it is so important to use only natural products (page 116). Always read the label; otherwise one might be poisoning the body unintentionally.

Young women are sometimes bothered by acne. Natural vitamin E, *rosa mosqueta* and neem oil mixed together is said to erase scars, even old ones, on the face and body.

My body does not seem to need any other supplement at this particular time in my life. My goal is that one day, my body, mind and spirit will live in total harmony, and there will no longer be a need for supplements.

I personally tolerate only sub-acid fruits: apricots, cherries, nectarines, peaches, plums, pears, apples, organic red globe grapes and papayas. Sweet, dried, acid and citrus fruit (except lemons) do not agree with me. Being Type **O**, I understand the reason why. They are too acid-forming in Type **O**'s system, so in my case, I avoid eating them. I have no snack between lunch and dinner; but take 1 tbsp. of Bio K (liquid acidophilus) with a large glass of lemon water (alkalizing) as a preventative measure to keep my colon healthy.

I am a fast oxidizer, I metabolize my foods extremely fast and slow down this process by eating foods that contain calcium and fat along with the simple carbohydrates such as found in fruits. Vegetables are metabolized much more slowly. My body seems to need the calcium and the fat in the yogurt and the sesame seeds to prevent me from becoming light-headed.

Keep in mind that Type **O** is not really a fruit-eater, but if eaten in moderation it will cause no blood sugar fluctuation.

Dinner at around 7:00 p.m. in wintertime consisting of a bowl of slightly steamed, organic vegetables, especially broccoli topped with 1/2 avocado or eggplant dip (page 106), 1/2 jar of homemade yogurt, and a homegrown yellow tomato or tabouli (page 106) and a glass of Vittel water.

Personally, I test all my food before eating. Food testing (page 115) revealed that carrots, celery, beets, lettuce and most sprouts do not agree with me at this point in my life.

In the summertime I eat lightly, some days just yogurt or soured milk with 2 tsp. spirulina added and a piece of seasonal fruit.

As mentioned, yogurt and soured milk are predigested protein and can be eaten at any time of the day, and are easily digested.

In the past I have tried many times to totally eliminate dairy and nuts/seeds from my diet, but so far I have been unsuccessful. At this point in my life I still need these foods to function properly. Being classified as a lacto-vegetarian is all right with me.

The last hour of the day I spend in meditation, thanking God for all the blessings received.

Chapter 10

IDEAL DIET FOR "A" BLOOD TYPES

Approximately 42% of the North American population is Type **A**. Research indicates that Type **A**'s are the descendants of farmers. The biochemical make-up of Type **A** is naturally made to be a vegetarian. Type **A**'s are highly intuitive with a sensitive body. In general, when balanced, they are calm, centered and everything they do is usually done in a harmonic way. Due to their calm and centered personality Type **A**'s operate on a low but steady energy, which indicates a lesser need for protein.

Type **A** in general can get all the protein needed to maintain a balanced body from the vegetable kingdom.

All animal products, such as meat, poultry, fish, seafood, as well as dairy products and eggs are all too mucous-forming in the Type **A** and should be totally avoided. The same usually applies to whole-grain products, which are too acid-forming. As mentioned earlier, if grains are desired, they should be sprouted. In the sprouting process the grains become more alkaline, therefore, less acidic (page 70). Soya beans are the only legumes recommended for Type **A**; all others are again too acid forming. The selection of vegetables should also be on the alkalizing side, preferably eliminating the acid forming ones such as red tomatoes (yellow tomatoes are less acidic), eggplant, red and white cabbage and sometimes even avocados. All can be too heavy for Type **A**'s sensitive system.

Type **A**'s ideal fruit selection is classified as sweet and sub-acid fruits eliminating the acid fruit, such as kiwi fruit, strawberries, blueberries (in general, most berries), as well as citrus fruits (grapefruit and oranges). Sometimes bananas, mangoes and papayas can cause an allergic reaction. Testing food before eating (page 115) is recommended.

As mentioned previously, a balanced Type **A** has no need to supplement the diet. The only exception being *probiotics* or homeostatic soil organisms (HSO) as a preventative measure to keep the colon perfectly healthy.

However, when supplements are required, I recommend herbal formulas (page 117) and natural food supplements derived from spirulina, blue green algae or "Pure Synergy," naturally grown vitamins and minerals (page 119). I also recommend any of the green grass juices.

Homeopathic remedies are also a good way to supplement, since they are mostly derived from plant sources, avoiding glandular extracts, derived from animals, and extracts suspended in alcohol. The reason for this avoidance is that alcohol is converted into sugar, which may aggravate the pathogenic (harmful) bacteria and cause yeast.

Again, I must emphasize how important it is to listen to your body and try to not upset it in any way.

The ideal exercise for Type **A** is definitely Yoga, which will keep the intuitive, sensitive body balanced and centered at all times. Yoga is the ideal stress release exercise for Type **A**.

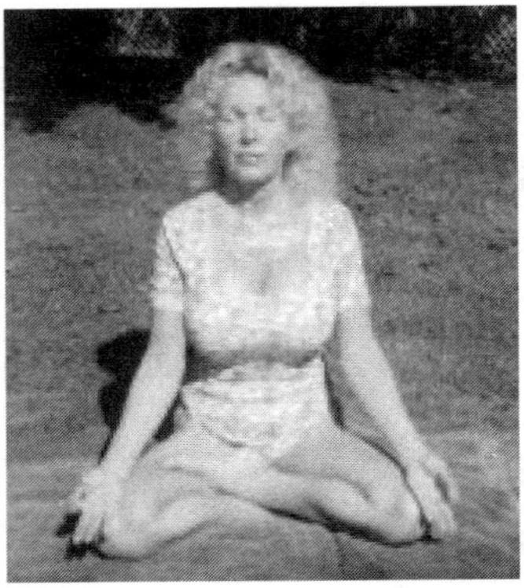

A comment on Yoga: I have been told by many Type **A**'s, that the blood type diet in conjunction with Yoga was the reason for their weight loss, a larger loss than one would experience on an average weight loss program.

Yoga is known to balance and realign the physical, emotional, mental and spiritual body when practiced on a regular basis.

Type A's Menu:

Breakfast:

- Cornflakes, oatmeal, buckwheat porridge with soya milk
- Sprouted millet/flaxseed (essene) bread with almond butter
- Rice cake with peanut butter
- Herbal tea such as alfalfa, ginger, or green
- Cashews/brazil nuts might cause an allergic reaction, test before eating, (page 115).

Snack: **(if needed)**

- Apples, apricots, cherries, grapes, peaches, pears
- 1 cup mixed-fruit tea
- Acid fruits such as kiwi, blueberries strawberries, and citrus fruits as well as banana, mango and papaya might cause an allergic reaction (test before eating, page 115)

Lunch: **(main protein meal)**

- Tofu vegetable stir-fry
- Tofu/bean burger on rye sourdough bread with sunflower sprouts (no wheat bread)
- Mixed beans soup with spinach salad and yogurt/hemp seed oil or tahini dressing (sesame seed butter and lemon water)
- 1 cup spearmint tea or filtered water

Snack: **(if needed)**

- Apple or cherry tofu pie
- Carrot/raisin cake made with spelt or hemp flour and flax/hemp oil
- Tofu or hemp ice-cream (in moderation only)

- 1 cup of peppermint or rosehip tea (works as a pick-me-up) or decaf coffee

Dinner:

- Lentil soup topped with soya cheese, mixed salad with garlic, lemon, virgin flax and hemp oil dressing
- Vegetable pizza topped with soya cheese (without red tomatoes)
- Fruit salad with plain *acidophilus* yogurt or carob tofu mousse (page 108)
- 1 cup fennel or chamomile tea
- Cabbage, eggplant, potatoes, red tomatoes, and beans such as; lima and garbanzo beans (chickpeas), (test before eating, page 115).

Avoid anything fermented or pickled with vinegar, especially if one has had Candidiasis in the past (page 74).

Chapter 11

IDEAL DIET FOR "AB" BLOOD TYPE

Approximately 4% of the North American population is Type **AB**. Research indicates that Types **AB** are the descendants of farmers and fishers, (a combination of Type **A** and **B**).

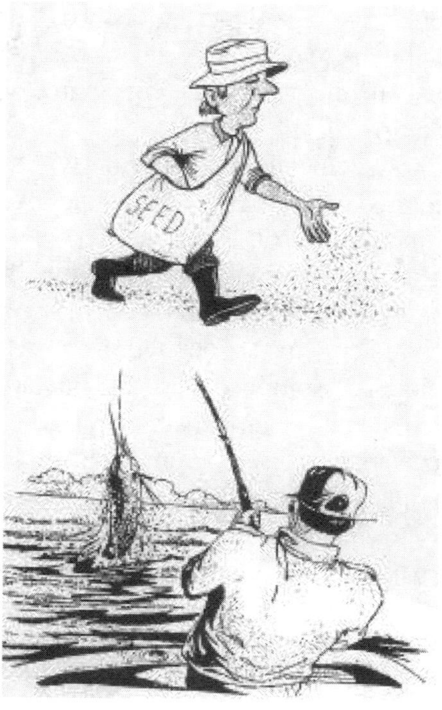

The biochemical make-up of Type **AB** is similar to that of Type **A.** In general, Type **AB** is even more sensitive and intuitive, with an alert mind.

Usually Type **AB** tends to be more active physically than Type **A**. Type **A**'s main nourishment should come from the vegetable kingdom.

For instance if one is not used to an all-vegetarian diet, a little fish may be added to the main meal of the day (lunch) once or twice a week, such as cod, trout, red snapper or salmon. However, stay away from: tuna, lobster, shrimp, mussels, or clams. Basically speaking, no seafood (or test before eating, page 115).

In general, meat and dairy products are also mucous-forming in Type **AB** most of the time and might need to be eliminated altogether. As mentioned previously, the only exception would be *acidophilus* yogurt or soured milk added as a salad dressing or eaten with a piece of fruit. Usually the same applies to whole-wheat products. If one desires whole grains it is advisable to use only the sprouted variety and organic soya products instead.

In general, Type **AB** diet is similar to that of Type **A** or **B** with a few exceptions considering their uniqueness. Type **AB** can usually tolerate tomatoes (especially the yellow ones that are less acidic) when eaten in moderation; the same applies to eggplant and cabbage. However, they do not do well on avocados, artichokes and all pepper varieties. In general all other vegetables agree with Type **AB** (test before eating, page 115).

As mentioned previously, supplements may not be required at all by the Type **AB**, except *probiotics* and homeostatic soil organisms (HSO), taken as a preventative measure to keep the gut healthy. If one desires to supplement for specific health problems, it is advisable to use natural food supplements derived from whole foods, such as alfalfa, chlorella, spirulina and all green grass juices (page 119). Herbal and homeopathic remedies in tablet, pellets or in vegetarian capsule from plant-based sources may be taken avoiding the alcohol-based extracts.

Synthetic-derived supplements are in general cheaper but usually cause more harm than good, especially in a sensitive person. If synthetic supplements are taken over a long period of time, they can be deposited in the body, especially the liver, causing liver problems.

The ideal exercise for Type **AB** is walking, to release stress. It is wise to consider meditation on a regular basis to calm an easily over-stimulated nervous system. When blessed with an alert mind, one must provide harmonious surroundings to nurture a powerful mind, avoiding overexertion in any way possible.

Defining Meditation:

Meditation does not mean sitting cross-legged on the floor. Meditation is concentrating on something, focusing attention on one object such as listening to classical music or birds singing, watching the sun rise/set or praying. Praying is asking God; meditation is listening to God's answer, just by being "still" is what meditation is all about.

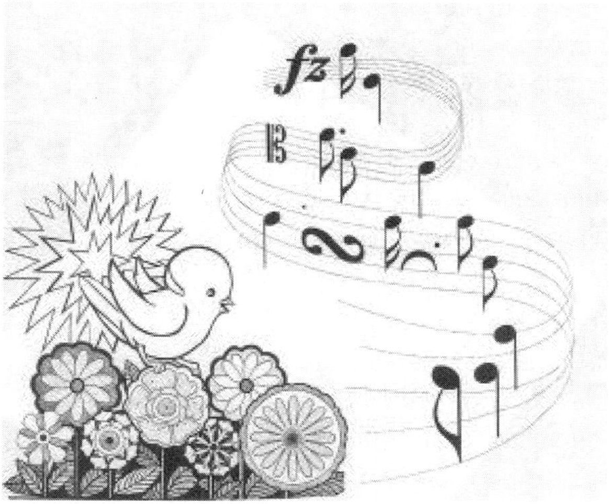

Type AB's Menu:

Breakfast:

- Millet or oatmeal porridge with Soya or rice milk
- Hemp granola with Soya or rice milk
- Rice cake with peanut, cashew or almond butter
- 1-cup of alfalfa or chamomile tea
- Hazelnuts, sunflower seeds and sesame seeds might cause an allergic reaction, (test before eating, page 115).

Snack: **(if needed)**

- Fruits such as apples, apricots, cherries, grapes, melons, nectarines peaches, papaya and pineapples.
- 1-cup mixed-fruit tea or spring water

Go easy on bananas, mangoes, citrus and all berries. You may want to eliminate them altogether

Lunch: **(main protein meal)**

- Bean/sprout/tofu stir fry
- Mixed sprout/tomato (yellow) sandwich with soya mayonnaise
- Fruit salad with 250 grams of yogurt
- 1-cup decaf coffee or green tea (acts as a pick-me-up due to containing some caffeine)

Snack: **(if needed)**

- Any fruit pie (using hemp/spelt flour) made from the above recommended fruit
- 1-cup spearmint or peppermint tea

Dinner:

- Mixed bean salad with basmati rice
- Millet/vegetable casserole topped with Soya or goat cheese
- Vegetable pizza topped with a few tomatoes (*preferably the yellow kind*) and soya or goat cheese
- 1-cup fennel tea or spring water
- Corn and buckwheat products, black beans, chickpeas (garbanzo beans) and lima beans, might cause allergic reaction (test before eating, page 115).

Avoid all fermented or pickled foods made with vinegar or yeast that can cause Candidiasis (page 74) in Type **AB's** sensitive body.

Albacore tuna or sardines may be added to the sprout and tomato sandwich, especially when on a transitional diet as well as flounder, sole, and seafood (test before eating, page 115).

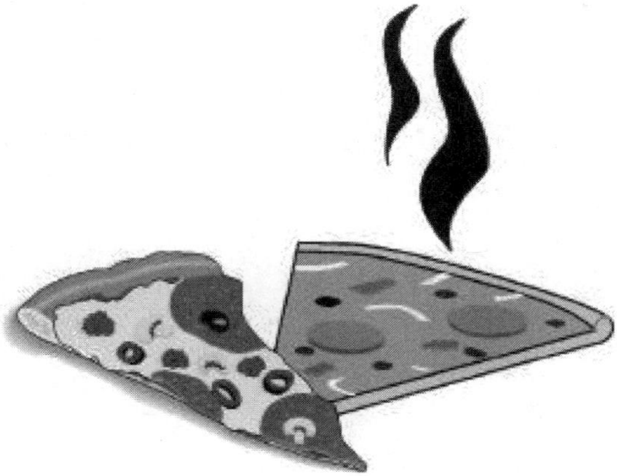

Chapter 12

IDEAL DIET FOR "O" BLOOD TYPES

Approximately 44% of the North American population is Type **O.** Research indicates they are descendants of the hunters.

Personally, I refer to Type **O** as the meat-eater (if they are 100% **O** and not a combination with another blood type). I believe that the Real Type **O** is the only blood type that can really tolerate meats (animal protein).

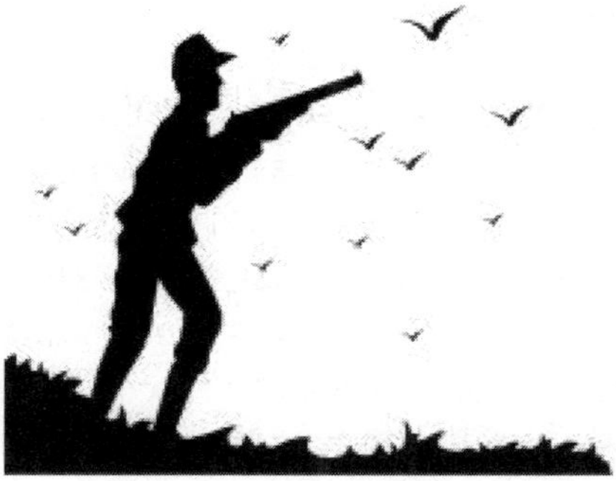

Type **O** has a high-energy body and therefore the need for protein is much higher than for **A** or **AB**. It seems that the Real Type **O** demands animal protein in most cases to function well (due to the **O**'s origin.) In general, the Real Type **O** cannot fulfill protein needs from the vegetable kingdom alone. However, there is always the exception to the rule. Considering parents' blood types can determine your real needs. Keep in mind to listen to the body to fully recognize its needs (testing food before eating is advisable, page 115).

Another exception would be a history of kidney problems. In that case a low animal-protein diet would definitely be more helpful than a high animal-protein diet. In order for the kidneys to recover faster, a high-protein diet would cause an extra burden on the kidneys and therefore, slow down recovery. It is known that most of the Real Type

O's have problems with digesting carbohydrates, the so-called starches, sweets and fruits.

Even the good complex carbohydrates such as whole grains, nuts, seeds and legumes might cause a problem (such as gas bloating, diarrhea, intestinal infections) or even weight gain when eaten in excess.

The weight gain can also be related to a mineral deficiency such as chromium and zinc, which seems to be low most of the time in Type **O**. Both minerals are needed to properly digest carbohydrates.

Type **O**'s have a tendency to overexert on a daily basis. They take on more responsibilities than they can handle, while thinking that somehow they will tackle the situation. However, if being continuously in such pressure-packed situations, a person is unable to balance weight or lose extra weight. Any stress makes losing weight impossible, because the body usually uses the extra pounds as a buffer, unable to handle the stress otherwise. The moment one balances life by removing extra stress (such as wrong diet, a hectic schedule, etc.), weight balances itself; this is called survival instinct at work. The body is trying to protect itself in any possible way to eliminate stress.

For Type **O**'s, fish can be tolerated most of the time. However, I believe that the Real Type **O** is a meat-eater, not a fish-eater.

Butter is well tolerated, but should be used sparingly. For salads, vegetables and pasta use virgin olive oil and canola oil for broiling and grilling.

Most beans, except navy beans, may cause bloating and gas in the Type **O.** Beans are a good source of protein, but the starch in all beans might still cause a problem, especially when trying to lose weight.

If bothered by recurring Candidiasis (yeast infection, page 74), one must eliminate all vinegar and yeast products, as well as mushrooms, soya products, sprouts, sugars, and substitute all fruits with vegetables. Stay away from alcohol, which is converted into sugar in the body. Drink only filtered or purified water; otherwise one is constantly feeding the yeast in the gut and cannot expect to recover totally until dietary changes are made. Sometimes just drinking herbal teas or decaf coffees can cause a reaction in a sensitive Type **O**.

Eliminate all pasteurized dairy products and eat only plain *acidophilus* yogurt or soured organic lemon milk and occasionally a little raw milk cheese. It is recommended to take *probiotics* (with a glass of lemon water) a half-hour before eating to kill the yeast and restore the friendly bacteria in the gut to keep the yeast from spreading test food before eating (page 115).

Type **O** usually can tolerate some dairy products, but only in moderation. It is advisable to use partly skimmed milk products. Skim milk should be avoided, since a little milk fat is needed to properly absorb the calcium in the milk. Homemade yogurt, when made from organic, preferably non-pasteurized (raw) milk, can be made from whole milk, as explained earlier.

Eggs should be from free-range chickens, poached and eaten in moderation. If grains are tolerated, it is best to eat the sprouted variety; otherwise, they might cause gas and bloating, indicating that the grains are feeding the yeast in the gut. If this occurs, it would be advisable to take *probiotics* such as *acidophilus* (without FOS) a half-hour before eating. When eating whole-grain products, be aware of weight gain. If weight increases when eating whole-grain products, they should be eliminated.

Keep in mind the Real Type **O** diet should be high-protein, low-complex carbohydrate. In simple terms, meat (protein) and plenty of starchless vegetables is the most suitable diet for the Real Type **O**. Some Type **O's** (especially the combination ones) are able to substitute meat with organic cheese, yogurt and nuts/seeds.

Eat fruits only in moderation. Sweet fruits such as bananas, figs, dates do not agree with many Type **O**'s. Citrus fruits (except lemons), pineapple and strawberries might cause indigestion (heartburn) and are not tolerated well (test before eating, page 115).

In general sub-acids fruits are best for Type **O,** including apples, apricots, cherries, grapes, nectarines, peaches and mangoes, to mention a few.

Being a Type **O** myself, I have had negative experiences with fruit juices. I believe fruit should be eaten whole and not juiced. If for any reason a Type **O** decides to use fruit juices instead of the whole fruit (which is in general more slowly digested than the juice), the juice should be diluted 50/50 with purified water.

As mentioned, Type **O** is not able to get all nutrients from foods and might have to supplement according to stress level. If not a smoker or drinker, basic antioxidants such as: Beta-carotene, B complex and vitamin C, microhydrin and natural vitamin E (mixed tocopherol) with Selenium are usually sufficient.

If unable to reduce stress naturally, through working outdoors (e.g., gardening) or exercising on a daily basis, supplementing should be considered (page 17). Testing of supplements is recommended (page 115).

The most suitable exercise for Type **O** is physical work, such as gardening or any workout, which involves the whole body, such as aerobics, treadmill, martial arts and passionate spiritual lovemaking. This lovemaking is inviting God into the heart and the bedroom, loving unconditionally, able to fulfill each other's needs, so that the two become one with God.

Keep in mind that Type **O** needs exercise to keep weight off and to stay healthy and fit.

Type O's Menu:

Breakfast:

- 250-gram plain *acidophilus* yogurt
- 1 apple
- 2 poached eggs with 1 slice essene rye bread and a little butter
- Millet porridge, 2% milk, topped with prunes
- 1 cup spearmint tea

Oats and all-wheat and Soya products might cause an allergic reaction (test before eating, page 115).

Snack: **(if needed)**

- Carrot or celery sticks with a few nuts such as; pecans, almonds, walnuts or 1 piece of sub-acid fruit
- 1 glass filtered/purified water or green tea
- Peanuts, cashews and brazil nuts (test before eating, page 115).

Most of the vegetables agree with Type **O**'s; however, corn, potatoes, olive and mushrooms might cause an allergic reaction, (food testing is recommended, page 115).

Lunch: **(main protein meal)**

- Organic chicken, mixed salad with garlic/olive oil/lemon dressing.
- Grilled beef steak with mixed vegetables
- Vegetarian omelet, mixed salad, homemade yogurt dressing
- 1 glass filtered/purified water

Snack: **(if needed)**

- 1 piece of sub-acid fruit such as apples, apricots, pears, peaches
- 1 cup peppermint or rosehip tea, (works as a picker-upper instead of coffee)

Dinner:

- Steamed vegetables with wild rice sprinkled with small amount of flax/hemp seed oil
- Spinach salad with artichoke pasta and hemp seed oil
- Caesar salad with garlic, olive oil and lemon dressing, topped with feta cheese
- Glass of filtered/purified water

Natural vs. Commercial Meat

What distinguishes one animal from another animal? One of the factors used for animal classification is what an animal eats, i.e. carnivores, vegetarians, etc.

Meats are most beneficial to the human body when from animals that have lived outdoors, eating a natural diet, i.e., beef, fowl etc., raised on grass with some organic feed added. Usually the label will state organically raised or free grazing. This kind of natural meat usually has ascorbic acid added as a preservative instead of sodium nitrate. Sodium nitrate has been scientifically proven to cause cancer and other illnesses. The majority of store-bought meats are usually from animals, injected with antibiotics and steroids to fatten them more quickly.

I do not believe for a moment that it is safe or healthy in any way to consume such meat.

Chapter 13

IDEAL DIET FOR "B" BLOOD TYPES

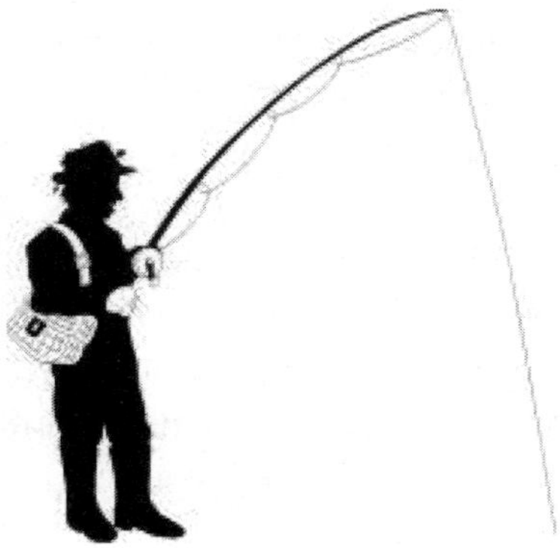

Approximately 10% of the North American population is Type **B**. Research indicates that Type **B**'s are mostly descendants of fishers.

I refer to Type **B** as the fish-eater. Type **B** shares the characteristics of both Type **O** and Type **A**. Type **B** should consider parents' blood type.

Type **B** usually has a medium energetic body due to being combination Type **A** (low energy) and Type **O** (high energy).

If one of the parents were a Type **O,** one would automatically lean more toward Type **O** characteristics. On the other hand, if one of the parents were a Type **A,** this would indicate they could easily be a vegetarian, if desired.

From my own experience, I believe one learns through trial and error. Listening to the body usually helps a great deal in such a situation.

Most Type **B**'s, have the same nutritional needs as Type **O,** except their protein supply should mainly come from fish and some seafood.

If one desires to become a vegetarian, this is the ideal diet to be used as a transitional diet.

Most Type **B**'s do not do well on poultry and meat. In general, complex carbohydrates usually do not cause a problem when eaten in moderation, this including sprouted grains, sourdough bread, whole-grain pasta and potatoes.

In general, Type **B** can tolerate dairy products well, especially organic, non-pasteurized (raw) milk products. This includes all kinds of soured milk; yogurt, kefir, lemon milk and mild cheeses.

I am usually not in favor of just drinking milk. Even raw milk is much easier digested when taken in soured form due to being predigested. This souring can be done by adding 1-2 tbsp. of fresh lemon juice to the milk; stir with a plastic spoon and enjoy.

Depending on the parents' blood type, soya products can either be tolerated or not at all. As mentioned, I am Type **OB** and unable to digest soya products. To satisfy unique nutritional requirements, learn to listen to the body (food testing is advisable, page 115).

Depending on one's occupation, physical activity and stress level, Type **B** might need to supplement on a daily basis. Sea vegetables such as blue green algae, chlorella, spirulina or green grass juices (page 119) are usually well-tolerated, when: Type **B** leans towards Type **A**; when Type **B** leans towards Type **O**, more antioxidants are required (details on page 18).

The best exercise for Type **B** is playing tennis and jogging in moderation. Avoidance of overexertion is important in Type **B**'s exercise regime.

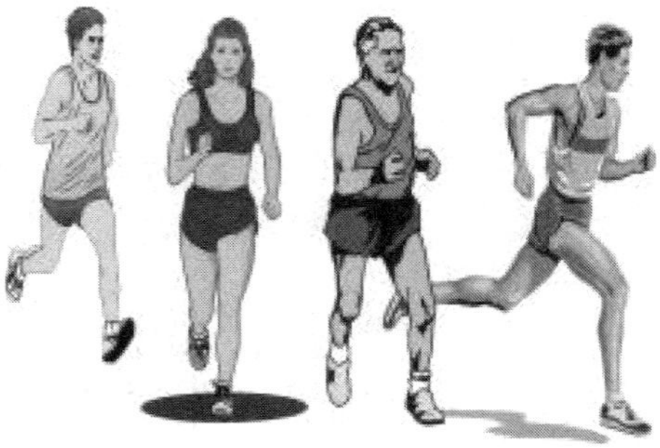

If Type **B** is out of balance and over-stressed, it is advisable to incorporate Yoga and meditation on a daily basis to rebalance the body, emotions, mind and spirit.

Type B's Menu:

Breakfast:

- Almond granola with almond milk
- Hot oatmeal with rice milk or milk
- 1 poached egg, yogurt and papaya
- 1-cup dandelion coffee with milk

Buckwheat and wheat products might cause an allergic reaction (food testing is recommended, page 115).

Snack: **(if needed)**

- 1 banana, grapes, plums in general, all seasonal fruits
- 1-cup of spearmint or mixed-fruit tea or just plain filtered water

Lunch: **(main protein meal)**

- Broiled fish such as cod, red snapper, trout or salmon
- Greek salad (topped with goat's cheese) with lemon/garlic/olive oil dressing
- Albacore tuna on whole rye, alfalfa and/or broccoli sprouts and soya mayonnaise
- 1-cup licorice tea or spring/purified water.

Clams, crab, lobster, mussels, shrimps, avocados, corn, olives, tomatoes (especially red tomatoes) and mug sprouts might cause indigestion or an allergic reaction (food testing is recommended, page 115).

Snack: **(if needed)**

- A handful of nuts (50 grams) such as almonds or brazil nuts, papaya or 1 apple and plain *acidophilus* yogurt
- 1 slice of fruit pie (made with hemp flour)
- 1-cup peppermint, rosehip, or green tea

Cashews, hazelnuts, peanuts and sunflower seeds, might cause indigestion (food testing is recommended, page 115).

Dinner:

- Mixed vegetables, cheese pizza without tomato sauce.
- Broccoli cheese soup, salad with yogurt or hemp seed oil dressing
- Vegetarian lasagna with soft cheeses and mixed salad hemp/flax/lemon dressing.
- 1-cup fennel tea or purified spring water.

Most beans are tolerated if eaten in moderation; if they cause indigestion, take *acidophilus* (1 capsule or 1 tbsp. Bio-K) after a meal with a cup of peppermint tea; this usually brings relief.

If bloating persists, Candidiasis might be the problem (page 74). A doctor's visit is recommended.

Chapter 14

DIFFERENT KINDS OF FOODS

Protein	**Starches**	**Fats**	**Veggies**
Almonds	Beans	Avocado	Asparagus
Brazil nuts	Breadfruit	Butter	Beetroot
Cashews	Buckwheat	Coconut	Broccoli
Cheese	Chestnuts	Olives	Spinach
Eggs	Corn	Pecans	Tomatoes
Fish	Lentils		Zucchini
Hazelnuts	Millet		Cabbage
Meat	Potato		Carrots
Peanuts	Pumpkin		Celery
Seafood	Rice		Cucumber
Sesame Seeds	Rye		Eggplant
Soya Beans	Sweet Potato		Lettuce
Sunflower Seeds	Wheat		Onions
Walnuts	Yams		Peppers
Wheat Germ			Spinach
Yogurt			Tomatoes
			Zucchini

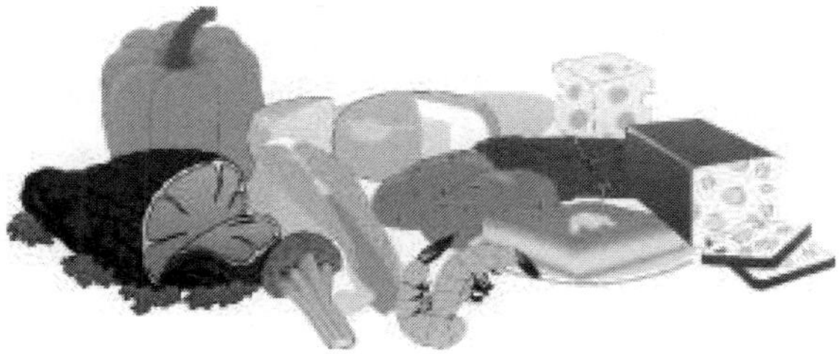

Different kinds of fruits:

Acid	Sub-Acid	Sweet
Blueberries	Apples	All dried fruit
Grapefruit	Apricots	Bananas
Kiwi	Cherries	Dates
Lemons	Grapes	Figs
Limes	Mangos	
Mandarins	Nectarines	
Oranges	Peaches	
Passion fruit	Pears	
Pineapple	Plums	
Strawberries	Papaya	

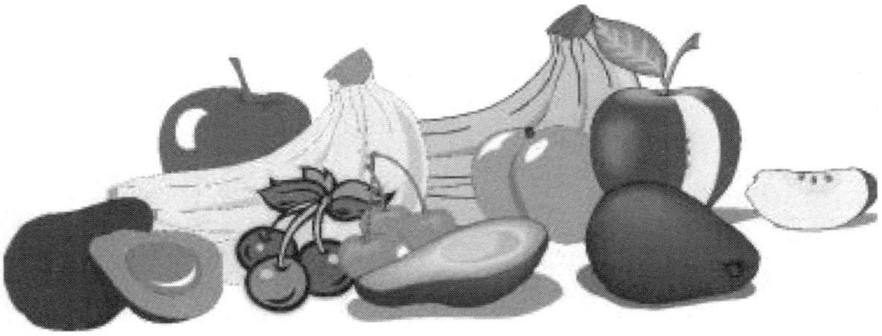

Chapter 15

DEFINING DISEASE

A diseased body is one that does not function with ease. The disease process begins when the body is unable to discard toxins through the bowels, kidneys, lungs, and skin in particular, the lymphatic system. Interruption in the removal of waste leads to lymphatic stasis (where the circulation of the lymph fluid slows down), which leads to further deposition of toxins and the beginning development of chronic disease.

For instance, when the body is injured or under attack by an infection, the lymphatic circulation is under tremendous strain, resulting in waste build-up. The result is swelling of the lymph nodes in the neck, armpits, groin, elbows and behind the knees. Therefore, it is of utmost importance to keep elimination channels functioning properly by drinking 6 glasses (1.5 liters) of water a day and eating in accordance with the blood type.

Personally, I recommend lymphatic drainage treatments, one session every three months to maintain a healthy body free of toxins. In an already-diseased body, two to four sessions per month are needed to assist the body in eliminating toxins and healing itself naturally.

There are two kinds of lymphatic drainage treatments available. One is through a registered massage therapist specializing in lymphatic drainage massage, the other is available usually through a holistic or alternative health practitioner using electronically assisted massage incorporating crystals and a high-voltage beam of photons.

Personally, I found the latter one the most effective tool in dispersing toxins and clearing the lymphatic channels naturally.

Chapter 16

ACID-ALKALINE FOOD CHART

Balanced body chemistry is of utmost importance for all blood types to maintain health and to correct disease.

All foods are burned (digested) in the body, leaving ash as a result of the burning process. This food ash can be neutral, acid, or alkaline, depending mostly on the mineral composition of the foods. If there is a depletion of the alkali reserve, one develops acidosis, or over-acidity in the tissues. For example: It takes 32 glasses of alkaline water to neutralize the acids from one can (12-ozs.) of cola. On the other hand, alkalosis (the opposite of acidosis), which is mostly seen in Type **O**, can be as detrimental to one's health as much as acidosis. Therefore, it is of the utmost importance that there be a proper ratio between acid and alkaline foods in the diet. Fresh lemon juice taken in water is most alkalizing. *Probiotics* are acid forming, which usually remedies alkalosis naturally.

1) The ideal ratio for Type **A** and **AB** is 80% alkali-forming foods, such as: vegetables and fruits and 20% acid-forming foods, such as: nuts, seeds, legumes and grains, to function best.

2) The ideal ratio for the Real Type **O** (the meat-eater) is slightly more acidic. The ratio is 70% alkali-forming foods mostly from vegetables with little fruit added, and 30% acid-forming foods mostly from meats.

3) The ideal ratio for the Type **B** is dependent on the parents' blood type, leaning more towards Type **A** or Type **O**.

Alkali-forming Foods

All fruits with the exception of cranberries, blueberries, and unripe fruit on a scale from 1 to 10 figs are the most alkalizing; all vegetables.

Neutral Ash Foods

Milk, butter, vegetable oils and white sugar.

Acid Forming Foods

All meats, eggs and most grains (with the exception of millet and buckwheat). Sprouted grains become more alkaline in the sprouting process.

Most nuts, seeds and legumes (except almonds and soya beans), when sprouted become more alkaline.

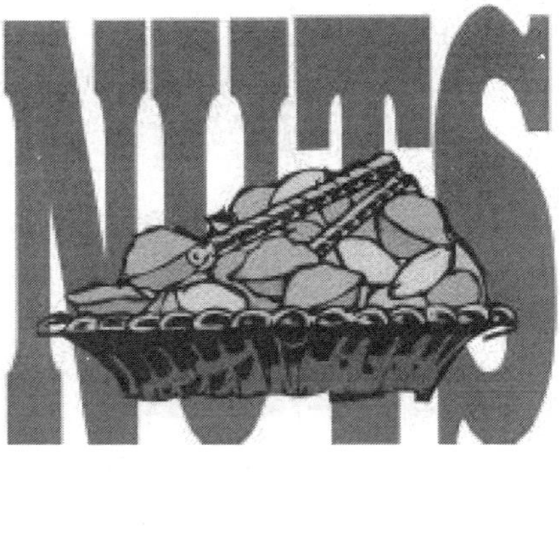

Chapter 17

AILMENTS: DISEASE AND BLOOD TYPES

Out of my own experience and research I have been able to relate specific illnesses to certain blood types.

Allergies: (food)

Food allergies can affect all blood types. Keep in mind that… One man's food is another man's poison, as James D'Adamo so nicely phrases it. There is a probability that food allergies could be reduced if we ate in accordance to our blood type.

Children can be especially sensitive to the chemicals in foods such as herbicides and pesticides when dealing with food allergies. Nowadays there is also a long list of chemicals, which are added to our daily food to give it longer shelf life. At this point we are not even considering what problems genetically altered food will cause in the long run. Many health authorities, including myself, believe that growing all foods organically would totally eliminate this particular food sensitivity. Eating according to blood type is strongly recommended to find relief.

A variety of herbal and homeopathic allergy formulas can be found in health food stores and pharmacies. I strongly believe one should not "self-prescribe". It is recommended to visit a certified/registered holistic health practitioner such as a naturopath, homeopath, nutritionist, or herbalist, for best results.

Type **O** might find more relief by adding bovine colostrums and homeopathic thymus glandular formula, extra Beta-carotene, vitamin C with bioflavonoids and microhydrin to the diet. However, emphasis should be placed on strengthening a weakened immune system by finding and eliminating the offender as the best solution (food testing is highly recommended, page 115).

Arthritis (osteoarthritis)

Most Type **O**'s (including myself) cannot digest whole grains especially wheat. If wheat is eaten over a long period of time, one can experience joint and other health problems due to the high acid content in the grains. Usually eliminating whole wheat will remedy the condition.

It is a widely accepted fact that fish, flax and hemp seed oils contain EFA's (essential fatty acids) that have an anti-inflammatory effect on joints. By eating plenty of slightly steamed vegetables and salads using flax/hemp seed oil as a dressing helps to naturally reduce the pain.

Types **A** and **AB** usually respond well to herbal formulas and homeostatic soil organisms (HSO) as well as applying topically devil's claw cream (Regime, page 117). Type **O** usually benefits from supplementing methylsulfonylmethane (MSM) and/or glucosamine sulfate, as well as elk velvet antler, colostrums, and salmon oil, plus vitamin C and vitamin E (mixed tocopherol.) These are also known to have anti-inflammatory properties. Coral calcium and magnesium oxide are known to reduce pain, as well as applying topically hemp/msm cream (Regime, page 117).

Medical research indicates that B12 stimulates bone cells called oesteoblats. Therefore, B12 is capable of regenerating bone. However, finding and eliminating the offender (by testing all foods and supplements, page 115) permanently strengthens the immune system.

According to Dr. Donsbach, when the pain is unbearable, adding 4 ozs. of 35% food-grade hydrogen peroxide to the bath usually brings relief.

Arthritis (rheumatoid arthritis)

It seems that Type **A**'s are more prone to rheumatoid arthritis than any other blood type.

I believe that in cases of inability to cope with stressful situations right away, all stress settles in the joints. Therefore, Type **A**'s responsibility is to create harmonious surroundings, whether at home or work. It is also well known that rheumatoid arthritis can be brought on by round worms that settle in the joints (a stool sample would confirm this possibility). If this is the case, using the "*Zapper*" (page 113) as directed will usually bring relief. At the same time it is advisable to adhere to an all-vegetarian alkalizing diet, concentrating on the more alkalizing foods such as vegetables and sub-acid fruits. It might also be beneficial to add alfalfa, spirulina, green grass juices and/or "Pure Synergy" vitamins/minerals (page 119) while eliminating grains, even the sprouted variety, until improvement shows.

Adding essential fatty acids (EFA's) to a salad such as flax and hemp seed oil (Hempola/Omega, page 117) is advisable since these supplements are known to have anti-inflammatory properties.

Other beneficial remedies are: Homeostatic soil organisms (HSO) and arthritic herbal formula. Beta-carotene and natural vitamin E (mixed tocopherols) have anti-inflammatory properties. Applying rain forest cream (Regime, page 117) topically usually helps reduce swelling. Homeopathy offers a great variety of remedies, tailored to an individual's needs.

Asthma

It is helpful when counseling people with asthma to know their blood type in order to be more accurate in recommending a certain diet or supplements. From my experience most of the time asthma sufferers are Type **A** and

AB. Food taken not in accordance with blood type can cause a severe asthmatic attack.

Offenders such as peanuts, wheat and pasteurized dairy products, are usually those that trigger breathing problems. By finding and eliminating (food testing, page 115) the one offender it is possible that you can restore your health.

In some asthma cases, especially in children, the cause could be parasites (worms). By eliminating the worms with the "*Zapper*" (page 113) in conjunction with the herbal parasite cleanse, usually eliminates the asthma as well. In a few people, asthma is not brought on by a physical problem, but an emotional one. Finding out what caused the emotional upset, and then resolving it, usually solves asthmatic attacks.

Helpful remedies are: homeostatic soil organisms (HSO), magnesium to relieve spasms, quercetin and manganese to stabilize cells. Applying to the chest a few drops of black caraway oil (Regime, page 117) helps to relieve spasms.

If no response occurs to any of the above, there might be a major health problem of which a person is unaware. In this case, it is advisable to see a specialist such as a holistic medical doctor, homeopath, or any alternative health practitioner. An organic vegetarian diet is highly recommended.

Candidiasis (yeast infection)

In my research, Type **O** seems to be most affected by Candidiasis. Type **O** is supposed to be a meat- and vegetable-eater on a high-protein, low-carbohydrate diet.

If Type **O** eats mainly refined carbohydrates over a period of time, one might be bothered by recurring yeast infections; even supplements are unable to cure it. A change of diet for a period of at least six months is recommended to give the yeast time to die out.

A healthy intestine normally houses a balance of friendly bacteria and yeast. Excessive sugar and alcohol consumption, excess use of birth control pills (use the natural approach instead page 117) allow an imbalance in the intestine as the friendly bacteria reduces in number. The yeast multiplies. The overgrowth of yeast in the gut or systemically (throughout the body) can be painful. A healthy immune system is capable of eradicating yeast, provided it is not growing too fast.

In the case of a classic yeast infection, *Probiotics* are needed to balance and re-establish intestinal flora. *Probiotics* should be taken as liquid (Bio-K), one whole container (100 grams providing 50 billion of friendly bacteria), upon arising on an empty stomach or before bedtime.

Helpful Remedies

The B-complex plus extra biotin should be taken preferably in capsule. The tablet variety needs binders and fillers to hold it together, which might also cause a problem especially in systemic Candidiasis.

- Ester C
- Quercetin
- Microhydrin
- Super halibut liver oil (A and D)
- Selenium oxide
- Zinc Citrate
- Garlic (preferably organic and fresh) oil
- Caprylic acid in capsule
- Colloidal silver as liquid
- Grapefruit seed extract (Ferlow, page 117)
- Natural vitamin E with CoQ10

Bovine colostrums powder or capsule (to strengthen the **O**'s weakened immune system) can be taken.

I am not in favor of encapsulated herbal formulas or alcohol-based tinctures for sensitive Type **O**'s. These supplements seem to worsen the condition. However, fresh plant extracts such as dandelion (Schoeneberger) to support the liver seem to be well tolerated. In severe cases Nystatin (Allopathic medicine) might be required which is available with a doctor's prescription at pharmacies.

In addition, cleansing the liver with fresh lemon juice (taken in warm water throughout the day) is most helpful, as are homeopathic remedies such as Nat sulph, Kali mur, Nat phos and candida.

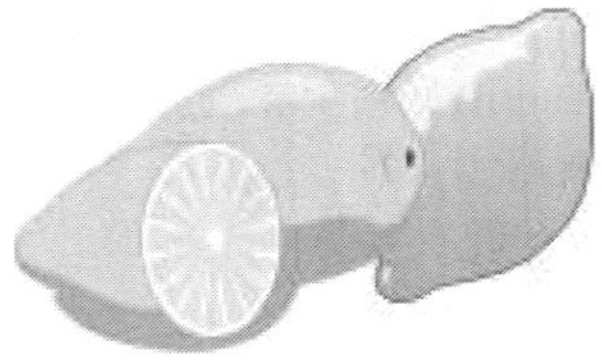

Most Type **O**'s have reported beneficial results when adhering to the blood type diet, taking the recommended supplements and using Dr. Clark's "*Zapper*" daily (page 113). Dr. Donsbach's oxygen therapy (adding to the morning bath, 4 ozs. of 35% food-grade hydrogen peroxide) will eliminate even systemic Candidiasis within 2 months. I highly recommend reading *Oxygen, Oxygen, Oxygen and "Hydrogen Peroxide*" (page 119), definitely a worthwhile try.

If Type **A** is bothered by Candidiasis, besides the wrong diet, the birth control pill is usually the cause (it would be advisable to replace the pill with LADY COMP, a natural contraceptive, page 117). The herb Pau d'arco and black walnut hulls taken in conjunction with dairy free *probiotics*, is usually sufficient to kill the yeast naturally.

Cardiovascular Disease

Contributing factors to cardiovascular disease include smoking, drinking alcohol, eating "junk food," lack of exercise and excess stress.

The Real Type **O** might be the only blood type, which is able to live such an abusive lifestyle. For the Real Type **O's** it is of utmost importance to change their lifestyle including an appropriate diet, eating according to their blood type to reduce further stress on their bodies.

The more sensitive blood types such as Type **A** and **AB** can develop cardiovascular problems due to being emotionally stressed; this includes the death of a loved one, a divorce or any emotional trauma, which involves the heart.

Keep in mind that we are not just a physical body. There is also an emotional, mental and spiritual body that cannot be visually seen.

Beneficial remedies are; Co-enzyme Q10, beta-carotene, ester C with bioflavonoids, coral calcium, magnesium oxide and natural vitamin E (mixed tocopherols plus selenium oxide). Other herbal remedies such as hawthorne berries, ginkgo biloba, and fresh organic garlic may be added to food. As well as essential fatty acids derived from salmon oil (for Type **A** and **AB** derived from hemp/flax oil), all are known to strengthen damaged arteries.

Homeopathic "rhus tox" is an emergency remedy to be used at the onset of a heart attack (to minimize the pain) until arrival at the hospital and can be taken up to one week after the attack.

Chicken Pox and Herpes Virus

Anybody can get chicken pox, but Type **O** seems to be more prone than any other blood type. Once contracted this virus remains for life, staying dormant in the body as long as one lives a balanced, harmonious and stress free life.

On the other hand, if exposed to stressors on a daily basis such as worrying about family, job or money, eating not in accordance with one's blood type, there can be an activation of the virus. One might wake up one morning with blisters in one spot or all over the body.

Most grains, nuts and seeds are high in the amino acid arginine. This particular virus loves arginine-rich foods to awaken and multiply, which explains why most grains, nuts and seeds awaken the virus.

On a scale from 1 to 10, pecans are the lowest and peanuts are the highest in arginine with seeds and grains in the middle. This virus loves chocolate and one might have to give up chocolate permanently to prevent further outbreaks.

To suppress the virus, lysine-rich foods should be added (to balance arginine and lysine), preferably eaten at the same meal. Lysine is mainly found in meat, fish, goats cheese, unpasteurized (raw) cheese, yogurt and mung beans. Lysine can be taken in capsules, each capsule providing 500mgs., three times a day.

Supplementing is helpful, but to gain permanent results the offender should be eliminated, avoiding nuts, seeds and grains to prevent further outbreaks (food testing is highly recommended, page 115).

To strengthen the immune system, sterols and sterolins seem to normalize immune function. Sterols can be taken in capsules (Moducare, page 118) or by adding organic milled flax seeds to a meal, but only if seeds are tolerated. The B complex and extra B12 may be taken sublingually or by injection for better absorption. B12 is needed by the nerves to maintain the protective myelin sheath, which is wrapped around nerves to insulate them. Super halibut liver oil, ester C with bioflavonoids, natural vitamin E with CoQ10 and zinc enhance immune function. Homeopathic remedies such as Echinacea and rhus tox are also beneficial.

Adding epsom salt (magnesium sulfate) and celtic sea salt (page 119) to one's bath and washing with liquid castile peppermint soap (page 116) help greatly to heal skin eruptions naturally. A topical application of one drop of lavender, tea tree and peppermint essential oil applied directly to the blisters helps to dry them out faster and healing occurs normally sooner. Some **O**'s recover faster when applying the above in conjunction with using the "*Zapper*" (page 113).

Constipation/Diarrhea

In general it is mostly Types **O** and **B** who are bothered by constipation (not eliminating within two hours after eating). Constipation is due to eating high-protein diets and not enough fiber from vegetables and fruit.

Types **A** and **AB** seem to be less constipated due to their higher fiber intake. On the other hand, if they are junk-food eaters, they might have the same problem as the Type **O**'s and **B**'s. It is of utmost importance to drink enough liquids, in general, 6 glasses (1.5 liters) of filtered water and herbal teas, as well as regulating the diet. Sometimes Candidiasis can cause either constipation or diarrhea. It is advisable to find, treat and eliminate the real cause and at the same time achieve regular bowel functions. Again *probiotics* are usually helpful in either the case of constipation or diarrhea.

Plain *acidophilus* yogurt eaten with prunes for breakfast in combination with 250 mgs. magnesium oxide and 300 mg. vitamin C (magnesium oxide and vitamin C are natural laxatives) usually remedies the problem. Changing diet is recommended if constipation is due to lack of fiber intake. Organic milled flax seeds and psyllium seeds may be added to plain yogurt followed by 12 ozs. of room-temperature, ozonated water (page 114) which usually relieves even stubborn cases of constipation.

I am not in favor of laxatives of any kind, even herbal ones; they all treat the symptom, but not the cause. Leading sedentary lives can also contribute to constipation. Any time anger, frustration or resentment constrict the body, it can result in chronic constipation in all blood types. Easy-going, happy, peaceful people are seldom constipated.

Edema (water retention)

Many overweight people are bothered by edema. Disorders that can cause water retention are heart and kidney failure; these need a medical doctor's attention.

The overweight Type **O** experiences edema when not eating according to blood type. Eating refined carbohydrates and not enough protein causes water retention and excess weight gain. Adhering to a high-protein and low-carbohydrate diet will prevent excess water weight. If Type **O** is deficient in either vitamin B6 and or vitamin C, they might also experience weight gain due to water retention.

Deficiency in potassium and excess in sodium are seen in Types **A** and **AB's** edema, due to mostly eating refined foods. An imbalance between potassium and sodium means that sodium increases and potassium drops. This condition can be remedied by eating a balanced vegetarian diet according to blood type, while focusing on vegetables and fruits that are high in potassium and low in sodium.

It is not advisable to take water pills, as they will not eliminate the cause of edema; only treat the symptom. Water pills have the tendency to remove the excess sodium as well as the potassium, thus, depleting the body. To achieve lasting results, the cause must be removed. Treating the symptom brings only temporary relief.

Fibromyalgia (muscle pain)

Fibromyalgia is most prevalent among people with Type **O** blood, the so-called over-achievers and perfectionists. Most of the time fibromyalgia is brought on by prolonged stress. Living a life out of tune with nature can lead to fibromyalgia. Symptoms are constant joint, leg and muscle pain. Your body hurts all over. Changing your lifestyle is a "must" to achieve permanent results (page 96).

The following supplements are recommended to minimize the pain:

- B-complex 50-100 mg.
- B12 1000 mcg. with folic acid 100 mcg (taken sublingually for better absorption)
- Microhydrin 1-2 capsules 250 mg.
- Natural vitamin E
- Selenium oxide 50 mcg.
- Co-enzyme Q10 50 mg.
- Ionized coral calcium (1-2 small packs a day)
- Magnesium oxide 500 mg.

The above supplements are taken with ozonated water (page 96) or quartz crystal energy water (page 120) at lunchtime.

If Types **A** and **AB** are affected with fibromyalgia, the likely cause is acidosis. It is recommended to consume more alkaline-forming foods (page 69) as well as adding green grass drinks to the diet to find permanent relief.

Some people feel pain all over their bodies. They believe they have fibromyalgia until a simple stool test (doctor's office) shows they are infested with parasites such as roundworms. In such cases, herbal parasite cleanse is recommended to naturally eliminate the parasites. At the same time, using the "*Zapper*" (page 113) may bring permanent relief. In the case of pets, treat them as well, to prevent re-infection by adding herbal parasite cleanse (black walnut hulls and wormwood, one capsule, more or less, depending on weight) mixed with their food.

Hypoglycemia

Hypoglycemia is caused by the over-secretion of insulin, resulting in an abnormally low level of glucose/sugar in the blood. When blood-sugar levels drop anxiety, irritability, panic attacks, mood swings or mental disorders are experienced. Research indicates that an overactive thyroid can also cause an increase in metabolism affecting the blood-sugar level.

There is great controversy among holistic doctors regarding diet; some recommend the high-carbohydrate diet while others, the high-protein diet. I believe by knowing your blood type, as well as that of your parents, provides the answer (food testing is recommended (page 115).

In general, Types **A** and **AB** can stabilize blood-sugar fluctuations with a high-complex carbohydrate, low-protein diet. Supporting the adrenal glands with the herbal formula (HIGL) usually minimizes stress on the body.

Types **O** and **B** can usually stabilize blood-sugar fluctuations with a high-protein, low-carbohydrate diet. The herb ginseng is helpful in normalizing body function by minimizing stress, as well as vitamins A, B, C, E, and magnesium. The trace mineral chromium is needed by all blood types to stabilize blood-sugar fluctuation.

As far as I know, apples are the only fruit, which stabilizes blood-sugar fluctuations in all blood types. The old saying; "An apple a day keeps the doctor away," is true. All blood types need to avoid all refined sweets, coffee, tea and alcohol, any one of which can trigger a hypoglycemic attack.

Insomnia

Insomnia is lack or loss of sleep. Type **O's** are most affected by insomnia. It is the executive-type Type **O**'s, "Superman" and "Superwoman," who are most bothered by insomnia. After a stressful day, working late hours, coming home late, they are unable to relax and enjoy leisure time.

If there are no physical causes to the problem such as parasites, it is recommended to change the lifestyle by incorporating walks in the woods or working in the garden.

Installing a "kiva light" (page 117) in the bedroom helps serotonin production, which turns to melanin at night, promoting better sleep.

The blood type diet is recommended, eliminating all proteins from the evening meal, such as red meats, nuts, seeds, garlic and onions. These foods are all stimulating and should only be eaten with lunch. Avoid coffee, tea, hot chocolate, as well as all stimulating herbal teas such as green tea, rosehip, and peppermint. Drink only plain unflavored, filtered water with a twist of lemon. Coral calcium and magnesium oxide each 500 mg taken with a glass of lemon milk (1 tbsp. of fresh lemon juice added to an 8 oz. glass of organic milk) taken before bedtime relaxes the body. To relax the mind, the homeopathic remedy coffea cruda is recommended.

If parasites are the problem, use the herbal parasite cleanse in conjunction with the "*Zapper*" (page 113) to find permanent relief. It is recommended to treat pets as well by adding herbal parasite cleanse (black walnut and wormwood,

1-2 capsules, depending on the weight of the pet) to their food to prevent re-infection. I use the above on my pets as a preventative measure, as it is known that parasites are transmitted from pet to owner.

Menopause

Menopause, or also known as "*the change of life*" is eventually and inevitably experience by all blood types. It is the start of a new phase in life.

Personally, I call it the beginning of the golden years and consider it absolutely nothing to be concerned about. The only change experienced is the absence of one's monthly menstruation, which is welcomed by most women. On the other hand, if the body has been abused in many ways, discomfort on a daily basis; such as hot flashes and mood swings, etc., may last for a few years.

I always knew turning fifty would be the trigger date for myself to stop menstruating; this is exactly what happened and all that happened. I experienced no discomfort whatsoever.

If bothered by hot flashes, taking 250 mg. of magnesium oxide and 200 iu. of natural vitamin E (mixed tocopherols) plus 25 mg. of vitamin B 6 with a little plain *acidophilus* yogurt brings to most women instant relief. This can be taken up to three times a day. In the case of diarrhea, one has taken too much magnesium and needs to adjust accordingly to bodily needs. Magnesium is a potent natural immune nutrient in which most women are deficient, especially during menopausal years. When the ovaries prepare to retire and the adrenal glands are supposed to take over, this adjustment can only occur when there is an ample amount of magnesium available to join with other minerals and trace minerals to be found in blue green algae, chlorella, dulse and kelp.

Magnesium oxide is also called the "cooling mineral." Magnesium is able to cool the body naturally.

Natural vitamin E (mixed tocopherol) acts as an estrogen substitute and is therefore capable of minimizing hot flushes, night sweats and mood swings. Vitamin B6 can raise progesterone levels, helping to correct high estrogen to progesterone ratios. A little yogurt eaten along with the above usually enhances the cooling effect. Magnesium and vitamin E and B6 can also be taken without the yogurt.

Some women find relief from applying natural progesterone and evening primrose oil to the skin a few times a day. Remember, you can learn through trial and error by getting more in touch with your body by listening to its needs (testing supplements is recommended, page 115).

Types **A** and **AB** might want to try the herbal menopause combinations especially formulated for menopausal needs. These formulas are beneficial through supporting the changing system. Some Types **A** and **AB**'s respond well to the herb derived from the chaste tree, called vitex. Vitex is known to balance estrogen to progesterone ratios when taken over a longer period of time. Black caraway oil (Ferlow, page 117) applied to the abdomen is known to relieve menopausal symptoms naturally. Homeopathic remedies such as belladonna, pulsatilla and sepia relieve hot flashes as well.

Some Types **O** and **B** might benefit more by adding to the diet magnesium oxide, vitamin E and B6, the total B complex, 50 mg., as well as 500 mg. of vitamin C with bioflavonoids and microhydrin 250 mg.

I am not in favor of synthetic Hormone Replacement Therapy (HRT). However, if a person gets satisfactory results, then this might have been exactly what was needed to feel better.

Multiple Sclerosis

Multiple sclerosis (MS) is caused by a virus similar to chicken pox and Type **B** seems to be mostly affected by it. This virus, to which one might have been unknowingly exposed in childhood, stays dormant in the body, causing no harm until later in life. When the immune system is stressed to the limit, due to stresses such as a hectic out-of-balance life, or food intake not compatible with the blood type, the virus might flare up producing neurological disorders. It is also believed, that mercury from dental metal, which is constantly released in the mouth and not excreted by the kidneys or bowels might contribute to MS. Residues from pesticides in food can also cause MS.

To strengthen the immune system, benefit maybe derived from the following remedies: Bovine colostrum (powder or capsule), the antioxidants A, B, C, natural vitamin E (mixed tocopherols) with selenium oxide and microhydrin, plus plant sterols/sterolins in capsule, or obtaining them through adding milled organic flaxseed meal and hemp nuts to the diet, 1 tbsp. three times a day.

Medical research indicates that MS in some cases is related to a B12 deficiency. When B12 is not taken sublingually or by injection it might not be absorbed. Magnesium oxide is a relaxant and a powerful immune nutrient, which calms the nervous system naturally. The herb St. John's wort is also well known for its healing properties to injured nervous systems. The homeopathic remedy Kali phos strengthens the limbs and back. Adhering to an all-organic diet such as the anti candidiasis diet (page 74) is most helpful, including *probiotics* no matter what blood type. A visit to the dentist is recommended to remove metal dental fillings, replacing them with resin/plastic fillings.

Nephritis (kidney infection)

Most of the time Types **A** and **AB** are bothered by kidney infections due to high animal-protein intake. Usually their systems are not accustomed to digesting animal protein, and this causes an extra burden on the kidneys. If there is no other reason for the infection, a vegetarian diet will bring great relief. In general, taking *probiotics* in combination with organic garlic (freshly squeezed) usually clears up the infection.

For recurring infections due to nutrient deficiencies, vitamin A from lemon grass, natural vitamin E (mixed tocopherol) and buffered vitamin C with bioflavonoids might be needed. Bladder/kidney herbal formulas may help to restore the proper function of the kidneys. Supplements may have to be alternated to see from which one the body benefits the most (testing supplements, page 115).

Kidney problems can also be brought on due to emotional trauma, since the kidneys and heart (as mentioned previously) are the seats of unresolved emotions. A variety of homeopathic remedies are available in health food stores. However, I am not in favor of self-prescribing homeopathic remedies; they are supposed to be administered by a homeopath or an alternative health practitioner familiar with the principle of homeopathy for best results. Homeopathic remedies are the perfect tools for emotional problems and when administered properly bring to the surface past hurt and pain to be released. Therefore, homeopathy helps resolve emotional problems in a safe and gentle way by balancing body, emotions, mind and spirit naturally.

When pain is unbearable, berberis vulgaris is the remedy.

Pernicious Anemia (Megaloblastic anemia)

Medical research indicates vitamin B12 is required by the body to make DNA, the cells' genetic material. A shortage of B12 will lead to impaired cell production.

Extreme fatigue, irritability, memory loss or light stomach pains might indicate a B12 deficiency. In such a case a medical doctor's visit is recommended. B12 injections may be used to keep the condition under control. The other alternative would be to take B12 sublingually for proper absorption. In general, B12 is added to the B complex;

however, if the capsule is swallowed, the B12 might not be absorbed at all.

Pernicious anemia, also called megaloblastic anemia, is mostly found in Types **A** and **AB**, when living on refined carbohydrate diets with little or no vegetables. It is most helpful to change the diet and at the same time, take food supplements such as spirulina and chlorella (page 22). Spirulina and chlorella are sea vegetables which have the highest B12 content as does the beneficial bacteria called homeostatic soil organisms (HSO), has twice as much as beef liver. Taking B12 in conjunction with folic acid sublingually might also be required, especially in the beginning to stabilize the anemic condition.

If Type **O** is diagnosed with pernicious anemia, bovine colostrums, *probiotics*, kelp and B12 with folic acid taken sublingually is recommended to stabilizing the condition.

Psoriasis

This particular skin disorder is mostly found in Type **O**'s. The skin rash might affect any part of the body, even the nails. I believe attacks are triggered by inadequate diet, exposure to stress on a regular basis, as well as excess fat (especially the hydrogenated kind) in the diet.

When Type **O**'s eat excess grains and dairy foods, their fat intake increases. Most Type **O**'s require a low-fat diet (most of the time being slow oxidizers, meaning, they burn their food too slowly) to function well. As we all know, stress of any kind leads to disease. By eliminating the above causes, most of the time the skin heals itself.

Type **O**'s usually benefit by adding essential fatty acids (EFA's) derived from salmon oil to their diet. Super halibut liver oil with vitamin D, natural vitamin E (mixed tocopherol), buffered vitamin C with bioflavonoids and the B complex as well as *probiotics* for proper digestion and assimilation of food may also be taken. According to Dr.

Donsbach adding 4 ozs. of 35% food grade hydrogen peroxide (page 119) to the morning bath helps heal the skin.

If Types **A** and **AB**'s are bothered by psoriasis, relief can be found by adding essential fatty acids (EFA's) derived from organic virgin flax/hemp seed oil 1-2 tbsp. two times a day plus the beneficial microorganisms (HSO) in capsules to the blood type diet. Applying topically, and alternating rain forest, chickweed or neem cream (Ferlow page 117) supports the healing process of the skin.

Homeopathic remedies such as arsenicum and graphite, as well as, natrium muriaticum might also bring relief. These remedies can be altered to discover which remedy works best. However, I believe that only a homeopath is able to select the most appropriate remedy for a person's unique biochemistry.

Ulcers (stomach)

Stomach ulcers can occur anywhere along the gastro-intestinal tract and are usually the result of stress. Any blood type can develop ulcers if exposed on a regular basis to stressful situations. However, Type **O** seems to be most bothered by ulcers due to always living life on the edge.

In general, Type **O**'s have a tendency to neglect taking proper care of their bodies. They usually take their health for granted and are most surprised when the body rebels and strikes back with illness.

It is well known that any state of anxiety triggers acid release in the stomach and prevents ulcers from healing. It is of utmost importance to alter lifestyles so the ulcers have time to heal. In some people the bacteria Helicobactor pylori might also cause stomach ulcers. This particular bacteria attacks people with weak immune systems.

By visiting underdeveloped countries and drinking unclean water, a person might be exposed to the H. pylori bacteria. This bacterium settles in the gastro-intestinal tract, where it causes discomfort such as diarrhea and ulcers.

If after altering your lifestyle, the stomach ulcers remain, one might need to consider taking the H. pylori blood test. If the results are positive, the medical doctor will usually prescribe antibiotics.

There is also a less-drastic approach available to kill the H. pylori bacteria permanently.

Beneficial Remedies

- Organic grapefruit seed extract has effective anti-parasitic, antiviral and antibiotic properties (Ferlow, page 117
- Colloidal silver, which controls inflammation and renews the lining of the stomach.
- Wild oil of oregano has anti-viral, anti-fungal, and antibiotic properties (page 120).
- Bladder wrack, a seaweed, is able to inhibit H. pylori multiplication.
- *Probiotics* are useful in inhibiting pathogenic (harmful) bacteria in the gut.

To support the immune system and heal the ulcer, it is recommended to take the basic antioxidants such as super halibut liver oil (A and D), B complex plus extra B12 taken sublingually. Medical research indicates that B12 helps people who suffer from viral and bacterial diseases recover faster, when 2000 mcg. are added to the B complex. Beta-carotene, buffered vitamin C, natural E (mixed tocopherols) with selenium, and especially zinc are all known for supporting wound healing.

Types **A** and **AB** benefit by adding Licorice DGL (deglycyrrhized licorice but only the DGL kind). Licorice DGL and slippery elm bark taken before a meal help to heal the stomach lining.

Using the "*Zapper*" (page 113) with the above, most of the time brings permanent relief.

The homeopathic remedy Natrium phosphoricum reduces the acid in the stomach after eating and also helps minimize stomach pain. Again, these remedies might have to be alternated to discover which remedy works best (testing supplements is recommended, page 115).

Vaccinations

Most parents are not sure if vaccinations are really needed for their children's health. There is great controversy regarding vaccines. Some are in favor, claiming vaccinations prevent epidemics and viral diseases, while others state that the outbreak of epidemics were on the decline before the introduction of vaccines.

Some doctors link diseases such as allergies, multiple sclerosis and chronic fatigue syndrome to vaccinations.

Medical research indicates that the chicken pox and small pox vaccines carry a variety of viral contaminants such as the herpes virus.

The above might not affect some people at all, due to their having a very strong immune system, however, some might not be so blessed.

Personally, I am not in favor of any vaccination due to a bad experience in my past. The small pox vaccination did not agree with me at all and caused many health problems during childhood. I believe knowing how to apply homeopathy saved my life from more misery.

Homeopathic remedies such as Thuja, Variolinum and Silica can counteract the negative effects of the vaccine, even when a person was vaccinated 30 years ago. One question arises: "How is it possible to reverse a vaccination given 30 years ago?" Remember, all is energy and energy can be rearranged.

The books, *Vibrational Medicine* and *The Cure For All Diseases*, explain in detail how energy (electricity) can be used to eliminate bacteria, viruses and parasites in minutes.

Once the cause (stressor) is eliminated, the body is able to heal itself.

Chapter 18

BLOOD TYPE SUMMARY

I hope that this information presented on blood types will help you to get to know yourself better. I am fully aware that I am perhaps presenting a new concept to the reader, one not widely known here in North America.

The blood type approach has been well known in Europe for the past 100 years. So far the approach has been very accurate with its information.

I believe the time has come to try a new concept. Not everyone needs to eat the same diet or take the same supplements to stay healthy, especially when remembering a person's biochemical uniqueness. You should at least give it a try before discarding it as just another "fad" diet.

Before recommending new health ideas, I have always tried them on myself for an extended period of time. I now recommend the "Blood Type Diet" and strongly believe that it is a worthwhile concept that might change your life for the better.

Before engaging in any dietary changes, it is advisable to ask your family physician if you are healthy enough to do so. If you decide not to try the "Blood Type Diet," at least you have read about it and are able to discuss it, should the topic ever arise.

I also believe that knowledge is power and therefore the key to "freedom." This belief means that you should accumulate as much knowledge as possible and apply this knowledge to yourself, getting to better know your God-given body and His needs.

You are then able to share this knowledge with others who might be in need of it. Knowledge is only good if shared with others. Knowledge kept to yourself is knowledge wasted.

In the *Old Testament*, Hosea 4:6, God said: "My people perish due to lack of knowledge." In the *New Testament*, Jesus shared His knowledge with those eager to hear it. In Luke 4:23, He said, "Physician, heal thyself," but this is only possible when the physician knows how to heal.

Sometimes a person might be instantly healed by God's grace and unconditional love for His children. But this is not meant to be for all; it depends on that person's purpose.

Remember, each one of us came here to fulfill a unique purpose. You must try with all your heart to figure out what that purpose is and then live up to it, so that your life will never be without a goal.

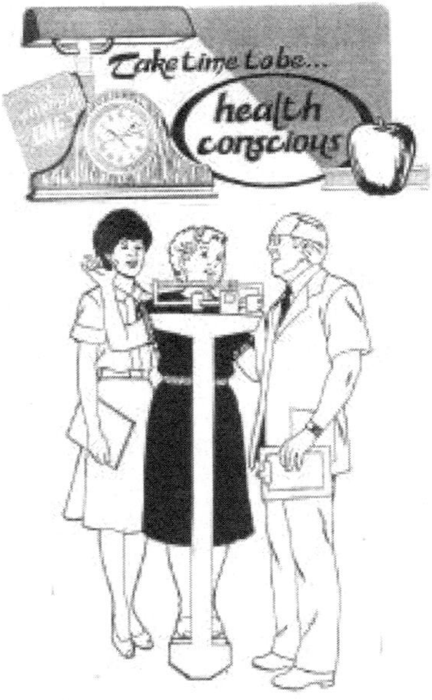

When I read the books; *From Enoch to the Dead Sea Scrolls* and shortly after, *Pythagoras*, teachings of the Greek philosopher who lived in 500 B.C., I knew what my purpose was. The only thing I did not know at the time was how to fulfill it.

Over the last few years I have asked God for guidance which I have received, revealed to me step-by-step. It takes faith to believe that we are not here by accident but that each one of us plays a unique part in the overall picture for the betterment of all of humanity. With that in mind, and God's blessings, "I wish you well."

Chapter 19

DO'S AND DON'TS FOR STAYING HEALTHY

Avoid	Use Instead
All genetically-altered foods	Organically grown foods available in health food stores, some food stores and from nationwide growers. www.cog.ca; www.organicgrowers.com
Herbicides, pesticides	Natural insecticidical soap of potassium salts of fatty acids (Safer's page 118) or 3% H202 or molasses (page 118)
Chemical weed control	Natural fatty acids (Safer's "TOP GUN" (page 118)
All hydrogenated fats: refined oils/margarine contain plastic materials (can be deposited in arteries)	Unrefined oils: virgin olive, hemp, flax, sesame (Hempola or omega, page 117) and butter
All vinegars in foods: Use only for cleaning carpets, windows and household appliances.	Lemon juice (alkalizing, and adds vitamin C to foods)
All soft drinks (sodas) too acidic.	Water filtered, purified, ozonated
Bottled water– can be contaminated with benzine (can cause allergic reactions)	Crystal energy drops (one drop per 1 oz.) to purify (page 118) or ozonate (page 114).

Avoid	Use Instead
Tap Water	Quartz crystal water filter (page 120), carbon countertop filter. For the whole house an ultraviolet sterilizer
Store-bought lemonade	Water filtered, purified, add lemon juice and raw honey
Pasteurized milk	Organic raw milk add lemon juice or vitamin C, purifies and curdles milk
All artificial sweeteners such as Aspartame and Saccharine are harmful (cancer-causing)	Stevia or honey
Table salt sodium chloride lacks minerals	Celtic sea salt contains 80 minerals needed by the body
Cooking pots/cutlery aluminum, stainless steel	Glass pots and plastic cutlery
All commercial cleaners laundry detergents, softeners, dishwashing liquid, floor cleaners, etc.	Natural biodegradable cleaners; laundry cleaners, borax, magnetic balls. Fresh lemon juice to remove stains
BHT and BHA synthetic preservatives that cause liver/kidney damage	Natural vitamin E d tocopherol or mixed tocopherols
Nitrates to preserve sausage and meat	Vitamin C citric acid
Monosodium glutamate (MSG) found in most Chinese foods, causes severe allergic reactions	Natural herbs/spices

Avoid	Use Instead
Bleach	Hydrogen peroxide (H202), lemon juice
Dry cleaning	Wash cloth with biodegradable detergent
Clothes dryer	Hang clothes in fresh air and sunshine
Carpet cleaner	Vinegar "vinegar plus", diluted
Wall-to-wall carpet	Wood or ceramic tile accent carpets should be washable; clean outdoors with diluted "vinegar plus" and brush
Wallpaper	Natural paints
Fluorescent lighting depresses immune system	Full spectrum, light, plant grow light or kiva light (page 117)
Chlorine/bromine in pools	Hydrogen peroxide 35% food grade H202
Microwave ovens Body cannot eliminate these rays and they are cancer-causing	Stove/oven (old-fashioned style)
Soaps/shampoos: conditioners, foam bath, cosmetic products made with Imadazolidinyl and diazo lidinylurea, known to cause contact dermatitis	Soap: natural liquid castile, hemp, jojoba, avocado, rosa mosqueta, sea vegetable, herbal and vitamin-based products (available in health food stores (read the label)
Harsh detergents: Sodium laureth sulfate and sodium lauryl sulfate, can cause eye irritation, hair loss and allergic reactions.	Aloe Vera or citrus extracts

Avoid	Use Instead
Buyyl/ethyl/methyl and propyl parabens: used to inhibit microbial growth and to extend shelf life. Known to cause allergic reactions and are highly toxic	Vitamin E, A, C and grapefruit seed extract as well as essential oils
Propylene glycol a petrochemical mix, used as a humectant, known to cause allergic reactions	Vegetable glycerin jojoba oil, hyaluronic and lactic acid
PVP/VA Copolymer a petroleum-derived chemical used in hairsprays and cosmetic products, known to cause breathing problems	Flaxseed extract
Stearalkonium chloride used mostly in hair conditioners and creams, known to cause allergic reactions and eye problems	Natural extracts derived from proteins and herbs
Triethanolamine (TEA) used widely in cosmetics to adjust ph, known to cause allergic reactions and eye problems	Herbal-based extracts
Synthetic colors such as FD&C, D&C are cancer-causing agents	Natural colors such as beta-carotene
Synthetic fragrances made up of many different chemicals, known to cause headaches, dizziness, vomiting and skin irritation	Organic essential oils (aromatherapy) lavender, rose, jasmine, patchouli, sandalwood, orchid (Aromaforce, Frontier (page 116 and Aura Cacia)

Avoid	Use Instead
Heavy metals: aluminum, barium, lead strontium, tin and titanium found in store-bought cosmetic products and toothpaste	Make your own cosmetics (I do) or use organic products from "Aubrey (page 116), Ferlow" (page 117) or "Neem Aura Naturals" (page 116)
Pressed or loose face powder	Organic cornstarch Aura Cacia and Aubrey
Toothpaste (fluoride is a toxic metal)	Baking soda or a few drops lemon juice, or H202 or microbrite
Toothbrush	Soladey-2 cleans teeth with solar energy (no toothpaste needed)
All hair dyes	Natural vegetable dyes
Mineral oil, baby oil and Vaseline are by-products of petroleum	Sweet almond oil or Aloe Vera gel to remove eye make-up
Personal lubricants	Natural vitamin E oil
Isopropyl alcohol (rubbing alcohol) a harmful cancer-causing solvent	Witch hazel fresh lemon juice and hydrogen peroxide (H202)
All metal dental fillings (including gold) leak and can cause illness	Resin/plastic fillings
Birth control pills cause hormonal imbalances	LADY-COMP a natural contraceptive (page 117)
Metal eye glasses depress the immune system	Plastic eye glasses not the cheap injected molded kind. Buy quality

Avoid	Use Instead
Store bought dog food: When labels read: meat by-products, ethoxyquin, propylene glycol and is preserved with BTA and BHA instead of natural vitamin E (mixed tocopherols)	Homemade dog food: Add hot 2% milk to quick-cook oats. Stir, cover, let stand for 10 minutes to thicken. Add cooked chicken pieces, veggies, 1/2 tsp. ground flax seeds and 1/4 tsp. spirulina powder (opt.). Stir all and feed to the furry children. Add 1 drop of liquid chlorophyll to their water to purify.
Clothing especially underwear made with synthetic fabrics such as nylon, rayon and polyester. All synthetic fabrics prevent toxins from being eliminated through the skin	Clothing of cotton, hemp, silk and wool
Dull colors such as black, gray and brown depress immune system	Bright colors Wear rainbow colors: Monday – red Tuesday – orange Wednesday – yellow Thursday – green Friday – blue Saturday – indigo Sunday – violet or white which represents all colors

Chapter 20

HEALTHY AND VERSATILE

How to Make Yogurt

To make homemade yogurt, use a commercial yogurt maker or any other glass jar with a lid. The milk should be organic and at room temperature. Fill the glass jar(s) with the milk and add one capsule of *acidophilus* culture (remember, the kind without the FOS) or 1 tsp. of the liquid variety (BIO-K, page 116). Stir the milk with a plastic spoon and close the jar.

The next step is to turn on the oven light (a 40-watt light bulb) and place the jar(s) in the oven, leaving the oven light on overnight. The oven light will warm the milk over a period of 12 to 15 hours, enough to make the milk curdle. For example, if the yogurt is placed in the oven at 7:00 p.m., the yogurt would be ready between 7:00 a.m. and 10:00 a.m. the next morning. After the above process is completed, the finished yogurt should be refrigerated. The culture in the yogurt remains alive for about three weeks.

The fat content of the milk, when curdled and eaten as yogurt, does not affect the cholesterol level, because the fat molecular structure is altered by the active lacto-bacillus bacteria such as *acidophilus* and is no longer harmful to the body. However, if eating commercially sweetened skim-milk yogurt, the above does not apply.

I make yogurt on a weekly basis, sometimes up to ten jars. I use the empty glass jars from nut/sesame butter, which are usually 450-gram wide-mouth jars. My yogurt is delicious and I always make enough to feed the whole family.

The Versatile Lemon

Besides being my favorite fruit, the medicinal value of the lemon is an antiseptic, meaning, preventing sepsis. Fresh lemon juice taken in warm water acts as a medicine, cleansing the system from impurities and helping the liver to detoxify. Lemons are useful in treating a cold, cough, sore throat, influenza, fever, heart burn (alkalizing the acid) and scurvy, to mention only a few possibilities on how to use lemons.

Lemons are high in potassium, calcium and magnesium as well as natural vitamin C. I use one lemon a day either to sour milk or mix the fresh juice with 1 tbsp. of tahini (ground sesame seeds) and eat it at lunch or dinner with yogurt. Sesame seeds are especially beneficial in liver disorders because of their high methionine content and calcium plus unsaturated fats. This combination cleanses and nourishes the liver. Most illnesses are the result of a toxic liver, so it is recommended to try the above and for faster results add the herbal liver cleanse formula (HEPA, page 119). Organic red beet powder (Frontier, page 117) combined with fresh lemon juice and tahini is an excellent liver food.

I use lemon juice and sunshine to remove stubborn stains and to whiten clothes. Lemon juice removes ink and rust stains as well as liver (age) spots from hands or face.

After gardening or feeding the dogs, I use lemon juice to wash my hands; it also takes away the odor from cutting onions and garlic.

The Versatile Hemp Seed

Hemp seeds are one of my favorites and are the most versatile seeds available. Hempseeds can be eaten as nuts, sprout them, or use the oil as a moisturizer and shampoo. Even clothing can be made from this substance.

Hemp seeds were a staple food to ancient civilizations. Now that it is legal to grow hemp in Canada and the U.S.A., it seems that humanity has rediscovered this ancient, versatile seed and its many uses. Hemp seeds are nutritious and high in protein (23%). The dehulled version of the nut contains 30% amino acids, essential fatty acids (EFA's), fiber plus vitamins such as vitamin E, carotene, B3 and B6 and minerals such as magnesium, zinc and iron. Its medicinal uses are limitless, since hemp has anti-inflammatory properties.

The health food store offers many different hemp foods such as hemp breads, muffins, cookies, milk and even ice cream. Hemp cookies and ice cream are a great natural healthy snack for children. If there is no health food store in your neighborhood, call: The Cool Hemp Company (Canada) (613) 757-3044. They will be pleased to send you samples of their all-natural organic hemp cookie, ice cream and nuts.

Sprouting Process (for seeds, nuts, grains and legumes)

The sprouting process is quite simple. In the evening place 2-3 tbsps. of organic seeds, nuts, grains or legumes in a wide-mouth glass jar. Rinse and cover with filtered or purified water. Cover with a cheesecloth and let stand overnight. Rinse every morning and evening for 2-3 days. Fresh organic sprouts are an enjoyable food.

To learn more about sprouting and the benefits of eating sprouted grains, seeds, nuts and legumes, I recommend reading:

The Biogenic Revolution by Dr. Edmond Bordeaux Szekely.

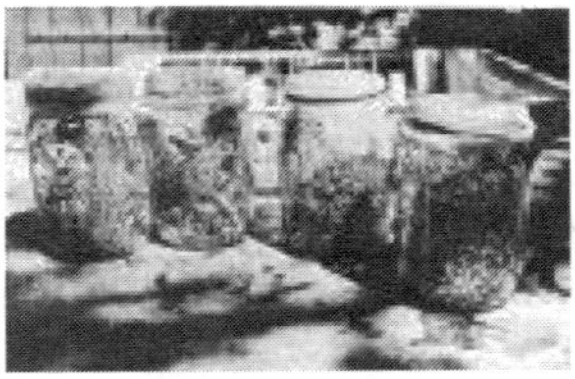

Chapter 21

RECIPES

During our stay in Cairo, Egypt we learned how to prepare Middle-Eastern dishes. Middle-Eastern cuisine is prepared from "scratch" with all natural, mostly organic ingredients. I call this type of cooking. "Vegetarian delight cuisine," especially suitable for Types **A** and **AB** (the vegetarians). If allergic to tomatoes and eggplant, substitute with other veggies such as cucumbers and zucchini. Type **B** might want to add laban (all-natural cream cheese). The Real Type **O** might want to add meat to the vegetarian dish. If allergic to chickpeas (garbanzo beans), substitute navy beans. Following are a few of my families' favorite recipes:

Humous (chickpea dip)

2 cups organic cooked or sprouted chickpeas
2-4 cloves garlic
1-cup organic tahini (sesame butter)
1/4 cup fresh lemon juice
1/2 cup finely chopped parsley
1 tsp. cayenne pepper (paprika), (optional)

Sprinkle finished dip with virgin olive oil. To make avocado dip, use the above, adding one avocado.

Soak organic chickpeas overnight. Drain off soaking water. Place in a stockpot, cover with 4 inches of water over beans. Cook 1-2 hours with garlic until tender or use canned organic chickpeas (EDEN FOODS).

Mash (or use processor) cooked chickpeas with enough bean liquid to create a smooth dip. Add remaining ingredients and mix well. Serve with celery/carrot sticks and/or organic unsalted corn chips (Que Paso or Bearitos) and/or pocket bread.

Baba Ghanoush (eggplant dip)

1 large eggplant (preferably organic)
1 clove garlic
1/2-cup organic tahini (sesame-seed butter)
1/2 tsp., cumin
1-2 tsp. Fresh Lemon Juice
1/4-cup chopped parsley

Trim and skin eggplant; steam till soft (approx. 10 mins.) Drain any excess liquid. Mix all ingredients well, chill and serve with organic unsalted corn chips or pita bread.

Tabouli (parsley/tomato salad)

3 diced tomatoes (preferably yellow and organic) or cucumbers.
1-cup finely chopped parsley
1/2-cup bulgur (cracked wheat) or substitute with wild rice, if allergic to wheat.
1-2 tsps. fresh lemon juice
1-2 tbsps. virgin olive oil

Mix ingredients together and serve. Nice topped with sliced avocado.

Falafel (bean patties)

2-cups organic cooked or sprouted chickpeas
1/2-cup organic cooked cracked wheat
2 cloves crushed garlic
3 tbsp. parsley
1 tbsp. virgin olive oil
1/2 tsp. cumin
1/4 tsp. black pepper
1/4 tsp. turmeric
1/4 tsp. coriander

Mix ingredients and shape into small patties. Bake in oven until golden brown.

Vegetarian Millet Gumbo Ba Tahini

4 cups organic kidney beans
1 onion
1 stalk organic celery
5 organic carrots
4 organic yellow peppers
2 garlic cloves
1/2 tsp. cayenne pepper
1/2 tsp. celtic sea salt
1 bay leaf

Soak beans overnight. Drain off soaking water and place beans in stockpot. Cover with 4 inches of water. Cook 1-2 hours until tender.

Sauté vegetables. Add cooked beans, spices. Stir and serve over cooked millet. Top with tahini sauce, sesame butter, lemon and a little water.

Laban (cream cheese)

Laban is made the same way as yogurt (page 102). Substitute organic milk with organic 10% cream. To make instant 18% sour cream, add to 500ml the juice of one small lemon and stir with plastic spoon. Best eaten with tabouli or falafel.

Lamb Balls

1-1/2 lb. lamb
1 egg
1/2-cup finely chopped onions
1-cup cooked couscous (durum semolina)
2 finely chopped garlic cloves
1/4 tsp. all spice
1/4 tsp. nutmeg
1/8 tsp. cayenne pepper
1/8 tsp. celtic sea salt or table salt
1/8 tsp. black pepper

1/4-cup chopped parsley
1/4-cup chopped pine nuts
1/4-cup sesame seeds

Mix ingredients well and form into inch-size balls. Bake in oven at 375°F for 15 to 20 minutes. Serve over cooked couscous (durum semolina wheat), millet or wild rice, topped with tahini sauce, sesame butter and a little lemon and water)

Non-Dairy Dessert:

Carob Tofu Mousse

2 small pkgs. silken organic tofu
1 small pkg. firm organic tofu
1-cup organic carob powder
1-cup fructose or 1/4 cup stevia
2 tbsps. natural vanilla
1-cup organic smooth almond butter

Mix ingredients well in food processor. Serve in champagne glasses or any attractive glass dish.

Apricot Delight

2 small pkgs. silken organic tofu
1 small pkg. firm organic tofu
1-cup organic dried apricots
3/4-cup organic smooth almond butter
1 tbsp. natural vanilla

Mix ingredients in food processor and top with fresh apricots. Serve in an attractive glass dish.

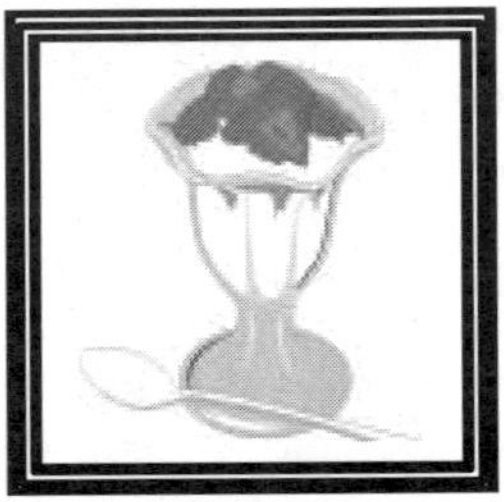

Chapter 22

MAKING SAFE COSMETIC PRODUCTS

Facial Scrub (to exfoliate dead skin cells)

2 tbsp. organic oatmeal
2 tbsp. organic ground flax seeds
2 tbsp. organic ground almonds
2 tbsp. organic rosehip powder (Frontier, page 117)
1 tbsp. jojoba oil (Aura Cacia/Now Foods, page 116)
1 tbsp. organic virgin hempseed oil (Omega, page 118)
2 tbsp. organic calendula oil (St. Francis, page 119)
2 tbsp. organic aloe vera gel (Nature's High, page 117)
2 tbsp. vegetable glycerin (Frontier, page 117)
1 tbsp. sea vegetable powder such as kelp, bladder wrack, dulse or irish moss.

Add 4 drops essential oil of chamomile and lavender plus 2000 iu of natural vitamin E (mixed tocopherols). Open gel caps and add to the above as a preservative.

Mix all ingredients. Put in sealable glass jar. Store in the refrigerator. The scrub is mild enough for daily use. The mixture can also be used as a mask. Put a small amount of scrub in the palm of your hand, add 1 tsp. of *acidophilus* yogurt to it mix well and apply to face/neck (avoid eye area) in a circular motion. Let dry for 10-15 minutes. Rinse off with warm water, follow with cold water, and apply toner.

Toner (tones and tightens all skin types)

Use organic aloe gel (Aubrey, page 116) or the kind in a brown glass bottle). Pour about 1 tsp. into the palm of your hand. Add 1/8 to 1/4 tsp. of fresh lemon juice (depending on skin sensitivity) and apply to face and neck (avoid eye area). Let dry.

Day-Time Moisturizer (all skin types)

As a cream base, use 4 ozs. shea butter (Frontier), also known as karite butter, a natural sun block, available in most health food stores.

Add to shea butter the following ingredients:

1/4 tsp. organic avocado oil (Aura Cacia, page 116)
1/4 tsp. organic apricot kernel oil (Aura Cacia)
1/4 tsp. organic rosa mosqueta oil (Aubrey, Ferlow, page 117)
1/4 tsp. organic jojoba oil (Aura Cacia)
4 drops essential apple oil (Frontier, page 117)
4 drops essential carrot oil (Frontier)
4 drops essential oil of chamomile (Frontier)

Open the gelcaps of 2000 iu natural vitamin E (mixed tocopherols). Add contents to the cream (acts as a natural preservative).

Blend ingredients and pour the finished product into a sealable glass jar. Store in a cool place (do not refrigerate). Use as needed by placing small amount in the palm of your hand. Rub palms together in a circular motion to liquefy. Apply sparingly to face and neck.

Evening Moisturizer

As mentioned previously (page 42), all I use as an evening moisturizer is 800 iu of natural vitamin E (mixed tocopherols) with a little organic virgin flax/hemp seed oil plus evening primrose and rosa mosqueta oil mixed together. I apply this mixture to my face and neck.

Body Lotion

Mix 2 ozs. unrefined organic grape seed oil with 2 ozs. unrefined organic jojoba oil. Pour into a brown glass bottle and preserve with 2000 iu of natural vitamin E (mixed tocopherols). Add a few drops of your favorite organic essential oil to the mixture and close the lid. Shake the bottle. Use sparingly. Store in a cool place.

Sunscreen **(not recommended for fair skin)**

To 2 oz. of unrefined organic sesame oil add 20 drops of essential oil of organic lavender, 2800 iu of natural vitamin E (mixed tocopherols) and 3 tbsp. of organic aloe vera gel. Pour into a brown glass bottle, close lid and shake well. Store in refrigerator. The mixture can be used before and after sunbathing.

When traveling, I alternate my homemade products with "Aubrey Organics" all-natural organic products that seem to be the only (store-bought) products agreeing with my sensitive skin and delicate hair.

If one would like to know more about natural organic skin and hair care, I recommend the book: *Natural Organic Hair And Skin Care*, by Aubrey Hampton. 1-800-282-7394.

Chapter 23

THE "ZAPPER"

The "*Zapper*," invented by Dr. Hulda Clark in 1988, is an electronic device capable of detecting and killing bacteria, viruses and parasites within minutes. It is simple, inexpensive, easy to use and it works (even when a person has been diagnosed as "terminally ill").

Once the cause of a health problem is eliminated, it is recommended to live a simple life in tune with nature and yourself, so the healing will last. Of the many healed, some returned to their old ways of living and their health once again failed. They had to start all over again.

To use the *Zapper*, one need not be ill. I use it as a relaxation and rejuvenation device on a daily basis. I meditate with the *Zapper* one hour in the morning and one hour in the evening. I find the best position is to lie on your back.

Place the *Zapper* (the size of a pack of cigarettes) on the solar plexus (navel area) and hold the copper pipes (covered with a wet tissue) on either side. Place the right foot on top of the left foot to create a circuit. It is known that the subtle energy flow of the *Zapper* removes blockages from energy centers (chakras), thus balancing, healing and rejuvenating the body naturally. During the one-hour session, refrain from wearing jewelry.

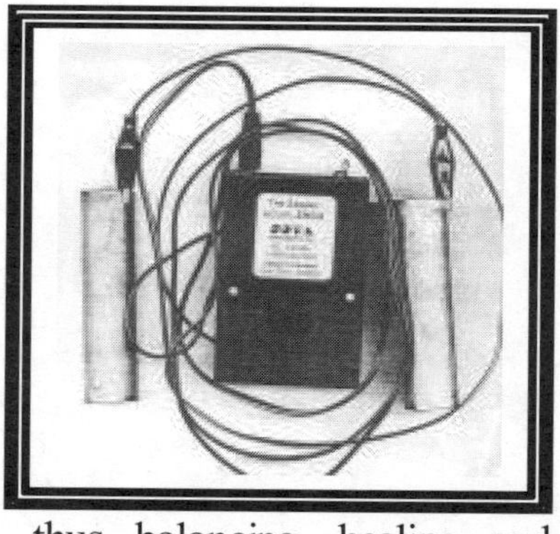

I experienced that my hair grows faster, wrinkles fade, and I look younger and feel great. If bothered by insomnia it is recommended to use the *Zapper* only in the morning.

The *Zapper*, and the book, *The Cure For All Diseases,* by Hulda Clark PhD., N.D., as well as the "ozonator" are available in Canada: Sota Instruments, 1-800-224-0242 or (250) 814-0046 and the U.S.A.: Self Health, 1-800-873-1663.

Chapter 24

Testing Personal Products and Food

All supplement quantities, personal hygiene, cosmetic products, medications and food. should be tested, either by applied kinesiology (muscle testing) or the "Omega Acubase System" (electrodermal acupuncture point testing). Both services are available through a holistic health practitioner such as a kinesiologist, nutritionist, homeopath, naturopath or a holistic medical doctor.

Be sure to take supplements, medications and foods needed by the body and which vibrate in tune with those unique vibrations. Personally, I hold (with both hands and standing) a supplement, product, or food on my solar plexus (navel), then ask my body if it is needed or beneficial to take and listen for the "yes" or "no" answer. Sometimes the life force (God within) bends the body forward (yes) or backward (no); that is all it takes to know. (*Touch for Health* by John F. Thie, D.C.)

After using the above method of testing for a while, just looking at a supplement, product or food, you will instantly know the answer.

When a person eats in accordance with their personal needs, not desires, then staying slim without counting calories or carbohydrates is an easier goal to attain.

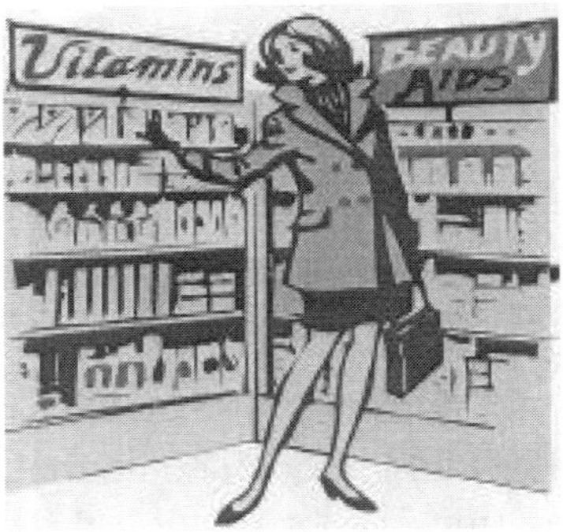

Products (store-bought)

TESTED FOR PURITY AND AVAILABLE FROM:

Aubrey Organics (U.S.A. and Canada) 1-800-282-7394: Natural organic shampoos, conditioners, hairsprays, body lotions, sunscreens, cosmetic and fragrances.

Aura Cacia (U.S.A.) 1-800-437-3301: Organic essential oils, body oils and cosmetics

Bioforce-Aromaforce (Canada) 1-800-265-0243: Organic essential oils (aromatherapy)

Bio-K (Canada) 514-954-1724: Liquid *acidophilus* 50 billion per 100 g., (dairy, recommended for Types **O** and **B)**

Carina Supply (Canada) 604-687-3617: Natural shampoos, conditioners, body lotions and hairspray

Chromalux (U.S.A) 914-698-1205: Full spectrum lighting

Dr. Bronner's (U.S.A) 760-743- 2211: Natural liquid castile soaps (peppermint-hemp)

Dolisos (Canada and U.S.A) 1-800-365-4767: Homeopathic remedies

Earthrise (U.S.A) 1-800-949-RISE, www.earth-rise.com: Certified organic spirulina powder/capsule, etc.

Ferlow Brothers *Regime* (Canada and U.S.A.) 604-820-1777: Natural organic shampoos, body lotions, medicinal oils, creams (black caraway, hemp/msm, rainforest, devil's claw, wild yam, tea tree, arnica, calendula, etc.) and organic essential oils

FoodScience (U.S.A and Canada) 802-878-5508: Vitamin B12 with folic acid (sublingual tabs)

Frontier (U.S.A) 1-800-669-3275: Organic herbs/spices, essential oils, shea butter, etc.

GreensPlus (Canada) 416-977-8765: Organic green food powder supplement

Hempola (Canada) 905-678-1066 www.hempola.com Organic hempoil, soaps, cosmetics

Infinity (Canada) 416-631-4000: Natural shampoos, conditioners and cleansing soap

Kiva Light (Canada) 1-450-226-3339: Healing light tube

Kroeger Herbs (U.S.A) 303-443-0261: Organic herbal formulas (capsule)

Lady Comp (Canada) 1-800-677-6699: Natural contraceptive

Nature's High (USA) (770) 889-8221: organic aloe vera gel

Natural Factor's (Canada) 604-415-4224: Vitamins (capsule) minerals, green powder. Probiotics (5.000 to 10.000 billions per capsule) and powder (dairy, Types **O** and **B**)

Nature Clean (Canada) 416-282-1107: Liquid Castile soap and biodegradable cleaning products

Nature's Way (U.S.A and Canada) 801-489-1500: Natural herbal formulas (capsule)

Now Foods (U.S.A) 708-545-9098: Organic foods, skin oils.

Omega Nutrition (U.S.A and Canada) 1-800-661-3529: Organic flax seeds, flax and hemp seed oil

Organika (Canada) 604-277-3302: Probiotic "Active *Acidophilus*" 5 billion per capsule (dairy free, for Types **A** and **AB**), herbs

Royal Body Care (U.S.A. and Canada) 972-893-4000: Microhydrin, microbrite, crystal energy drops

Purity Life Health Products Ltd. (Canada) 1-800-265-2615: Moducare (sterols and sterolins), and Kroeger Herbs

Safer's (U.S.A. and Canada) 416-291-8150: Natural insecticidical soap and weed killer

Simply Clean (Canada) 1-800-265-7245: Biodegradable cleaning products

Sisu Enterprises (Canada) 604-420-6610: Encapsulated vitamins and minerals

Soladey-2 (Canada) 1-888-825-5360: Solar energy toothbrush

Solgar (U.S.A) 877-276-5427: B Complex/vitamins (capsule)

Sprout Master (Canada) 705-322-2222: 35% Food Grade Hydrogen Peroxide (H2O2), Organic sprouting seeds, beans and grains, Organic Neem tree ("Aura Naturals"} skin care products and books:
Oxygen, Oxygen, Oxygen by Dr. Kurt. W. Donsbach
Hydrogen Peroxide by Conrad LeBeau
Advanced Tachyon products, etc.

Swiss (Canada) 1-800-268-9879: Magnesium oxide 420 mg. (elemental mag.252 mg.)

St. Francis Herb Farm, Inc. (Canada) 613-756-6279: Organic medicinal oils (calendula) and skin cream

Symbiotics (U.S.A and Canada) 1-800-784-4355: Organic colostrum powder and capsules

The Grain & Salt Company (Canada) 519-934-9948

Gold Mine Natural Food Company (U.S.A) 1-800-475-FOOD: Celtic Sea Salt

The Herb Works (Canada) 519-824-4280: Organic Herbs "HEPA"(capsule) and ointments

The Heritage Store (U.S.A) 804-428-0100: Edgar Cayce formulas, body oils and cosmetics

The Soap Works (Canada) 1-800-440-5597: Natural pet shampoo (repels fleas and ticks naturally and it even works.)

The Synergy Company (U.S.A) 435-259-5366: Advantage Health Matters (Canada) 1-800-338-6138: "Pure Synergy" Naturally organic grown vitamins, minerals and green drinks

Vibrant Health (Canada) 1-888-337-8427: Opal Essence Water Revitalizer (quartz crystal)

Wild Oregano Oil (U.S.A) 1-800-243-5242

WWOOF (Willing Workers on Organic Farms) (U.S.A.) offers free room and board in exchange for help. Some organic farms offer bed and breakfast. Call John at 250-354-4417

Chapter 25

AN INTRODUCTION TO "BAJARDIN"

If interested in knowing more about the Essene way of life (living in tune with all that is), the book, *From Enoch To The Dead Sea Scrolls*, reveals how to do so.

If you desire to live the Essene way of life, you may be interested in contributing your God-given gifts to the project called "Bajardin," meaning Garden of Baja. Bajardin is a holistic lifestyle project to be developed on 4000 acres on the Bay of La Paz, Baja California Sur, Mexico, facing the Gulf of California.

For more information on Bajardin, please contact: Rahmon Iturbe Henderson via

E-mail rahmoniturbe-@hotmail.com

TREE OF LIFE REJUVENATION CENTER

If you are interested in an established Essene Center, the "TREE OF LIFE REJUVENATION CENTER," founded by Gabriel Cousens M.D., would be the perfect place to familiarize yourself with what organic life, food and living the Essene way of life is all about. Personally, I recommend the center for Types **A**, **AB** and **B**. However, Type **O's** who are trying to switch from an all meat-eating diet to a vegetarian diet (even if it can only be accomplished for a week) will find the "TREE OF LIFE REJUVENATION CENTER" the perfect place to do so.

No matter what is experienced, you will always remember the breathtaking, tranquil setting of the TREE OF LIFE REJUVENATION CENTER, located on 166 acres in the Patagonia Mountains, Patagonia, Arizona. Phone (520) 394-2520. E-mail healing@treeoflife.nu/www.treeoflife.nu

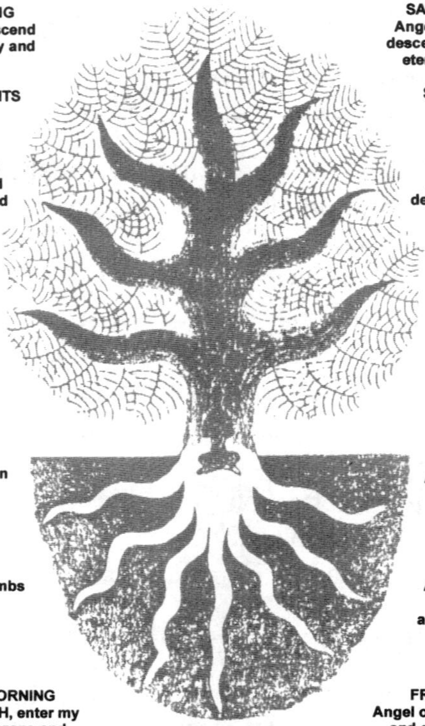

THE ESSENE TREE OF LIFE
With the Morning and Evening Communions

RECOMMENDED READING:

Blood Relations, Blood Groups and Anthropology
Ernest Arthur Mourant

You Are Your Blood Type
Naomi Toshitaka and Alexander Besher
(Out of print; library copy only)

Eat Right For Your Type
Peter J. D'Adamo, N.D.

One Man's Food... Is Someone Else's Poison
James D'Adamo

Blood Groups and Disease
Ada Kopec and Kazimiera Domaniewska-Sobczak
(Out of print; library copy only)

Character, Blood Groups, and Constitution
K. Fritz Schaer, M.D.

What's Your Type?
Peter Constantine

Traditional Foods are Your Best Medicine
Ronald F. Schmid, N.D.

What Your Doctor May Not Tell You about Menopause
John R Lee, M.D.

Colostrums, Life's First Food
Daniel G. Clark, M.D.

The Miracle of MSM
Stanley W. Jacob, M.D.

Clinical Homeopathy
Anton Jayasuriya

Stop Herpes Now
Barbara B. North, Ph.D., M.D.

Alkalize or Die
T.A. Baroody, Jr., M.D.

Encyclopedia of Natural Healing
Sigfried Gursche, M.H.

Oxygen, Oxygen, Oxygen
Dr. Kurt W. Donsbach, DC.,ND.,Ph.D.

Beyond Probiotics
Ann Louise Gittleman, M.S.,C.N.S.

Spiritual Nutrition, The Rainbow Diet, and Conscious Eating
Gabriel Cousens, M.D.

Vibrational Medicine
Richard Gerber, M.D.

The Living State
Albert Szent-Gyorgi

Star Gods: Clone Masters of the Universe
Brad Steiger

Twin Souls
P. Joudry and M. Pressman, M.D.

Recommended Reading:

The Biggest Secret
David Icke

Humanity's Extraterrestrial Origin
Arthur David Horn, M.D.

The Seat Of The Soul
Gary Zukav

The Bible Code
Michael Drosnin

The Bible
The Old Testament
The New Testament

1. The Essene Gospel of Peace and
2. From Enoch to The Dead Sea Scroll
3. The Essene Jesus
4. The Living Buddha
5. The Biogenic Revolution

Prof. Edmond Bordeaux Szekely
Available from:
I.B.S. International
P.O. Box 849 Nelson, B.C.
Canada V1L 6A5

PYTHAGORAS
Thomas Stanley
Available from:
The Philosophical Research Society, Inc.
3910 Los Feliz Boulevard
L.A., CA 90027

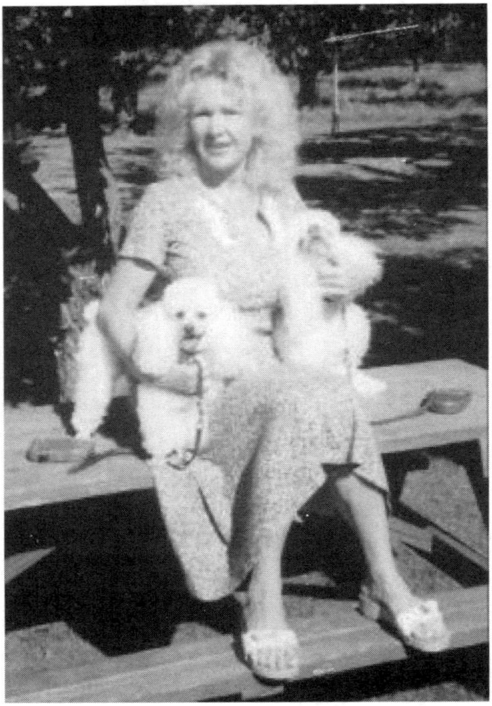

For each copy sold, 50¢ will be donated to Women for Women International, an organization fighting against *"female circumcision and equal rights for women."* For more information log onto:

- www.womenforwomen.org
- www.equalitynow.org/brochure
- www.rawa.org/contact.htm